Smoke and Mirrors

PETER DUFFY FRCS MD MBE

Whistle in the Wind was supposed to be a once-and-for-all-and-forever book. A cathartic release of pent-up frustration, a chance to heave over a particularly heavy and awkward NHS whistleblowing stone, expose the unfettered, corrupt and ugly truth and provide an opportunity for others to glimpse what festers beneath. Hopefully too, an opportunity to share what I have learned about speaking out from within a public sector monopoly employer, improve the chances for future whistleblowers and lay to rest the traumas, hypocrisy and double standards of the previous decade.

Completed without any editorial oversight in early 2019, the family spent months agonising over whether to publish or whether to simply leave it be; perhaps something to come back to and reflect upon in later years, or maybe an account for as-yet-unborn grandchildren to flip through in some far-off, still undetermined future.

Relatives and friends were clear that the text was both readable and relevant. Encouraged but terrified of further adverse consequences and retaliation, it took a full legal review to persuade me that publishing really was something I could undertake. Fiona and Edward sacrificed many hours correcting my typographical errors and we were ready to go by late July 2019.

But if I'd thought that publishing my account would both set things straight, and also mark an end to dirty tricks, spin, counter allegations, evidential tampering and both regulatory and investigatory inadequacies, I couldn't possibly have got it more wrong.

Peter Duffy.
Lancaster,
Christmas 2020.

Cover design by Gregoire Saul, Graphic Designer.
DaftCatStudio.co.uk

The second volume of Peter Duffy's enthralling account of his treatment by the University Hospitals of Morecambe Bay NHS Foundation Trust (UHMBT) is as compelling as the first. The book addresses the deeply disturbing and dangerous culture embedded in the NHS management at the UHMBT. This culture is persistent, deliberate, tarnishes the executive of the Trust and threatens the integrity of everyone who works there.

The Mid-Staffs Public Inquiry was chaired by Sir Robert Francis, an experienced medical negligence lawyer and veteran of the Bristol Royal Infirmary, GMC (General Medical Council) disciplinary hearing and appeal to the Privy Council. Sir Robert's contribution to UK Healthcare and the medical professions was 'a duty of candour', imposed on the healthcare professions, including hospital management, to honestly inform patients and their relatives of any adverse events occurring in their care and impacting their well-being.

The findings of the Mid-Staffs Inquiry were published in February 2013 and the 'duty of candour' added to the Health & Social Care Act 2008, by regulation, in 2014.

The inclusion in The Act introduced a statutory duty of candour for all healthcare providers in England to ensure that they are open and honest with patients when things go wrong with their care.

When Peter Duffy followed his professional obligations and duty of candour he had no idea where it would lead.

This book follows the truth and makes for painful reading as a healthcare professional and also as a possible NHS patient.

A must-read sequel to a very dark and as yet unfinished passage of NHS history.

Professor Stephen Bolsin. MBBS, FRCA, FANZCA, MHSM.

Previously Professor of Anaesthetics and director of the division of peri-operative medicine, anaesthesia and pain management, Geelong Hospital, Victoria, Australia.

Steve Bolsin is now the Executive Director of Medical Services and Clinical Governance for St John of God Health Care, a not-for-profit healthcare and social services provider in Australia and New Zealand.

Also, the consultant whistleblower for the Report of the Public Inquiry into children's heart surgery at the Bristol Royal Infirmary 1984-1995, an act of safeguarding which led to a full public enquiry costing £14 million and covering nearly 220,000 pages of evidence.

———————

An email from 2014, undiscovered by numerous freedom of information requests and purportedly sent by Peter, suddenly comes to light in 2020 and brings perilously close the end of Peter's fight to clear his name. Its impact is compounded by a lack of corroboration by those trusted with running NHS IT services and internal or external investigations. Will we ever know when, why, how or by whom this email was created, and will anyone be held accountable or has a dangerous precedent been set by all those involved?

Peter's book is an honest, engaging, emotional and troubling account of his ongoing challenges to defend his professional reputation and career. It gives insight and reflection on the involvement of patients, colleagues, witnesses, NHS management, government, regulators and the law in cases of retaliation against medical whistleblowers. It has uncomfortable parallels with the flawed Post Office trials, with misguided assumptions that IT systems and processes are reliable and secure, and the extent to which people will go to create or cover up evidence.

Ms Lucy Hunt. MEng (Oxon.), MSc Cyber Security (Lancaster University).

PhD whistleblowing researcher, University of Lancaster and IT consultant, with over 20 years work experience in the UK.

———————

I'm very sad to read that a referral to the GMC was used against Mr Duffy to try and counter the impact of the legitimate concerns raised by him.

The campaign 'Patients First' lobbied the health regulators, and as a result the GMC commissioned a review by Sir Anthony Hooper into malicious referrals in 2015.

He listened to our evidence and agreed that for doctors to feel empowered to raise patient safety concerns, their regulator needs to back them. It is tantamount to further bullying to have counter allegations of no validity sent to the regulator.

Sir Anthony recommended that the Medical Director of the employing Trust should confirm in writing whether a doctor has raised concerns prior to any referral. This tests the honesty of the Medical Director.

But disappointingly, this story confirms what many of us have learned.

The system is harming doctors who speak up, it is working against us (I hasten to add that the same goes for nurses, and others in health and social care).

Dr Kim Holt. Fellow of the Royal College of Paediatrics and Child Health.

Consultant Paediatrician and NHS whistleblower in relation to child protection and the death through child abuse of baby Peter Connelly (Baby P) in Haringey, London. 2007.

In 'Smoke and Mirrors' Peter Duffy has exposed the sinister, Machiavellian underbelly of parts of the NHS, its regulators and its political leadership.

The systematic mistreatment by UHMBT that resulted in his unfair dismissal as adjudicated by an employment tribunal was described in Whistle in the Wind. We might have expected that to be the end of the matter but in this, its sequel, he describes an intensification of the actions against him which are clearly aimed at destroying his professional reputation and any small chance of personal happiness that remained. This included forging an email purporting to be from him and which put him in the frame for a patient's avoidable death.

Read that sentence again.

The NHS claims to value whistleblowers and has an impressive array of mechanisms to ensure they are heard and not victimised. This narrative of Peter's experiences and his analysis of those experiences shows them all up for what they are. A sham. In 2014 I met Sir Robert Francis to discuss his Freedom to Speak Up Review, after he was commissioned by Jeremy Hunt, the Health Secretary. He promised to finish off what he began at Mid-Staffs and end the blood-sport of NHS-whistleblower pursuit. This book, along with the experiences of others, demonstrates the abject failure of his efforts.

Peter's last word is, 'When is this going to end?'

The answer, of course, is never. Unless someone with the political clout decides it will.

Dr David Drew. Ex-Fellow of the Royal College of Paediatrics and Child Health.

Consultant Paediatrician. NHS whistleblower and author of *Little Stories of Life and Death*.

One of the books that inspired *Whistle in the Wind*.

Patients' extraordinary trust in the NHS is founded on the expectation they will receive safe care when they are at their most vulnerable. But, too often, patient safety investigations describe known problems where staff felt unable to voice concerns.

Peter Duffy's integrity, motivation and resilience belies the personal cost of raising concerns to try to ensure patient safety. His story demonstrates the often-intolerable pressures. We have to do better in implementing a 'just culture', both for patients and for healthcare professionals for whom an unsafe working environment also results in harm.

We owe a debt of gratitude to Peter – one which extends to his wife and children, who have suffered consequences too.

Susanna Stanford. BSc.

Patient Safety and Human Factors Advocate.

When NHS leaders are allowed to attack and crush an NHS whistleblower, they are ultimately being allowed to attack and crush the public interest.

Peter Duffy exposes an entire industry that has built up on helping NHS leaders cover things up. Vast sums of public money are consumed by individuals skilled at undermining the public interest and depriving both NHS staff and patients of justice.

In my own case, 54,000 junior doctors were argued out of statutory whistleblowing protection to try and stop my case being heard (which succeeded for 4 years).

The NHS whistleblowing problem involves things like unaccountable power, money, misconduct and dishonesty. The various whistleblowing initiatives and champions are not brave enough even to acknowledge the actual problem, let alone propose a meaningful solution.

Peter Duffy's book does both, but is anyone listening?

Dr Chris Day. MBBS. Emergency Medicine Doctor and NHS whistleblower.

Following an open letter to Jeremy Hunt, Health Secretary, copying in 200 journalists, Hunt's office contacted our campaigning group of https://sharmilachowdhury.com/2014/06/03/letter-to-jeremy-hunt-2-help-justice-for-sharmila-chowdhury/

Sir Robert Francis, QC subsequently undertook the 'Freedom to Speak Up Review' which was published in 2015. Sir Robert made many recommendations including local guardians in every hospital and a National Guardian.

However, the local guardians are not independent and do not report to the National Guardian. They instead report to the local senior management. So, any raised concerns go to management.

Sad to see that despite taking part with this extensive review and campaigning for nine years, meeting with prominent ministers and heads of governing bodies, very little has changed.

Staff are repeatedly advised to raise any concerns and they will be protected. However, no protection exists, as none of the regulatory bodies, including the CQC, take raised concerns seriously. There have been instances where it has made whistleblowers' situations worse as the CQC end up telling the management.

Frequently, Trusts are left to investigate themselves i.e. mark their own homework. So, it is no surprise when they conclude they were unable to find any wrongdoing apart from a 'dysfunctional department'.

Not only are concerns not investigated, but whistleblowers find themselves being bullied which frequently follows false counter allegations, mainly to cover up the real concerns which have been reported, and to discredit the whistleblower. This leads to dismissal, with loss of career, pension, reputation, family union and even suicide as the only way to stop the ongoing nightmare. The whistleblower even starts believing the false narrative.

Organisations use public money in destroying the whistleblower, who has bravely reported concerns to protect the public.

There is an imbalance of justice. Organisations have ready access to legal funds, whilst whistleblowers, without a job and income, are frequently unable to challenge.

We currently do not have any regulatory body that takes whistleblowing seriously. When contacted by a whistleblower, they frequently advise they cannot get involved due to an ongoing legal process.

The very process, of course, which should not have been happening in the first place.

Currently, despite raising concerns, no lessons are learned, and so there are no changes or improvements and a continuation of placing lives at risk.

There needs to be an independent governing body that looks into concerns and also looks into the treatment of the whistleblower. Unless that happens, nothing will change.

During my campaign I discovered there needs to be some form of available help. So, I have created this website:

sharmilachowdhury.com

Sharmila Chowdhury. Imaging Services Manager, NHS &
private sector.
Previously superintendent for uroradiology at The Middlesex
Hospital, London (now UCLH) and NHS whistleblower.

----

*Peter Duffy's account of retaliation against his whistleblowing
reveals the way in which the whistleblower can find themselves
subject to a quasi-archaic testing of their endurance. A good deal of
what is inflicted on them feels punitive, even if it is not formally
recognised as punishment, which, of course, means there can be no
appeal against it.*

*Whistleblowers, like Duffy, take their stand on their commitment to
their organisation's professed values, and can sometimes then suffer
a sense of their moral world splitting in two as it becomes clear that
for certain purposes their organisation runs on quite different, if
concealed, principles. By those principles the whistleblower is
subject to a kind of punishment that is intended less to reform, than
to break them.*

*The alternative moral world in which whistleblowers then find
themselves is one in which their rights are frequently replaced by an
assumption of prior guilt, and in which instead of having access to
due process the whistleblower is trapped in a bureaucratic maze
whose tendency is to isolate, exhaust and demoralize them, prior to
their ejection not merely from the organisation they work for but,
where retaliation can effect this, from their entire professional life.*

Dr James Brown. Associate Research Fellow.
Birkbeck, University of London.
Joint co-ordinator of the BISR Guilt Group.
http://www.bbk.ac.uk/bisr/research/guilt-working-group/
https://soundcloud.com/user-642267037/
https://notthatjamesbrown.bandcamp.com/

Every day we as patients put our trust in the NHS to keep us safe. When something goes wrong we rely on clinical staff to speak up for us. The least we expect is that they are safe to do so. In Peter's first book, 'Whistle in the Wind', we hear just how difficult that can be and how anyone can be persecuted for doing the right thing.

It takes a very brave person to take on such a large institution that is prepared to do anything to silence those who are speaking up for patient safety.

In Peter's second book he lays bare the tactics that have been used to smear and discredit him because he refused to be quiet and go away. Persecuted just for doing his professional duty to keep us safe and not be silenced.

This isn't an isolated case. This has happened to many other clinical staff within the NHS, with their lives now ruined for doing the right thing for patients and their safety.

Peter's book 'Smoke and Mirrors' uncovers the relentless dirty tactics that are used against whistleblowers, and exposes a culture of fear, instead of safety. Until those that are part of and help to create this culture face serious consequences, sadly nothing will ever change.

Julie Bailey. CBE.
Principal whistleblower for the Mid-Staffordshire NHS Foundation Trust scandal.
Author of *From Ward to Whitehall – the disaster at Mid-Staffs*.
Founder of *Cure the NHS*.

'Give me six lines written by the most honourable person alive, and I shall find enough in them to condemn them to the gallows....'

'To know how to disguise is the knowledge of kings....'

'Secrecy is the first essential in affairs of the state....'

Cardinal Richelieu, 1585–1642.

Dedicated, once again, to the decades of commitment, quiet professionalism, values, sheer, over-and-above honest hard graft, and now sadly, the treasured memories of two of my most loved, committed and valued mentors:

Mr Bob Thomson FRCS. Consultant Urological Surgeon.
Mr Richard Wilson FRCS. Consultant Urological Surgeon.

R.I.P.

Well, you're cycling home from a long day at work in the pitch dark on your dirty, knackered old push-iron, heading back to your cold, empty and lonely flat. It's ******g down with sleet and rain, you're tired; in shorts, you're wet through, muddy and shivering and you've got about a third of the way home. And you think to yourself... 'is this really what I spent nearly four ******* decades of incredibly hard graft working towards? Surely nothing can possibly get any worse than this...?'

And then you get a puncture....

Peter Duffy. Facebook Messenger.
11th March 2020.

I was talking of this with a senior manager of a large multinational organisation. He laughed with a kind of ironic, pitying recognition and then said, 'This is just how it is in our large corporations; that's how they operate. You shouldn't be surprised, and you certainly shouldn't take it personally.... If I publicly challenged the ethos or strategy of my company I would be sidelined or eliminated very quickly. That would happen usually with great skill and stealth. How do they do it? Well, you'd best ask our HR or Legal Department—they're very good at it!' He smiled warmly, with a brief flash of strong white teeth. He was certainly right about large commercial corporations. It would be equally true in any dictatorship and any totalitarian organisation.

And it is what we are struggling with now, in our NHS.

Dr David Zigmond. Retired GP and Psychiatrist, London.
British Journal of General Practice, published January 2021.

Foreword

Amy Fenton

THE CONCEPT AND RELEVANCE of a whistleblower has become, sadly, all too common in today's society.

And yet, despite the important role such individuals can play in highlighting wrongdoing, correcting injustice and influencing policy, it is also a concept which deserves far more prominence in the media than it is currently afforded.

Because, for journalists, the industrial landscape has evolved to the extent where we are rarely given the opportunity – and, most importantly, the time, to direct our undivided attention to one single story.

Yet, when I first began speaking to Peter Duffy, I knew instantly that this was one of those career-making moments that most journalists can only dream of, and one which would require my full attention.

Over the last few years we have worked closely together, with the jointly shared ultimate ambition to improve patient safety, and to ensure that lessons are learned when mistakes are made.

Peter is an incredibly modest and unassuming individual who is reluctant to acknowledge the significant part he has played in highlighting the need for transparency and candour that our beloved NHS deserves. And to do that is the small part that I feel I can play in his incredible story.

I have often joked to Peter that, should I ever need the services of a urologist, he is the only person I would turn to, and I have said the same about his former colleague Richard Wilson, to whom this book is jointly dedicated.

Both Peter and Richard are perfect examples of what the NHS should be about, and the expertise the service should support and encourage, and yet the biggest tragedy through all of this is that the NHS no longer has either consultant providing the exemplary care that they are renowned for.

Throughout all my interviews and meetings with Peter's former patients I have always felt a sense of pride to hear how much he is respected and missed and it truly is nothing short of a tragedy that the NHS no longer has him at its disposal.

And although Peter feels his only option is to work outside the service, he continues to make a difference to patients on this side of the Irish Sea by ensuring that lessons ARE learned and that patient safety remains a priority for health bosses. And that is indicative of his professional dedication and integrity.

It has been nothing short of a privilege, and an honour, to be able to report on Peter's story and through it I have also made lifelong friends; not just with Peter himself but also with many of the patients and their families who have formed part of the saga we refer to as the urology scandal.

Amy Fenton,
Lancashire,
June 2021.

Prologue

SMOKE AND MIRRORS is darker, more complex and less accessible than *Whistle in the Wind* and, in the best tradition of sequels, will almost certainly underperform its predecessor; in sales, reviews, coherence and impact. However, I am determined not to use this as an excuse for inaction, particularly when there is the opportunity for much more honesty, learning, insight and safeguarding.

The recent international tragedies of the Boeing 737 Max crashes and, closer to home, the huge and entirely avoidable loss of life in the Grenfell Tower inferno have once again underlined the importance of encouraging a universal public duty of candour, safeguarding and respect for the safety and lives of others. Causing 346 and 72 entirely avoidable deaths respectively, no one can even begin to properly compute the scale of suffering, pain and emotional distress from these entirely unnecessary tragedies.

But compare these figures with the human and financial fallout from medical errors, harm, neglect and omissions.

Around the world and according to the World Health Organisation, nearly 140 million people every year suffer adverse events from unsafe healthcare.

Of these, over 2.5 million will be fatal.

This compares with a global average of about 300 fatalities per year from commercial plane crashes.

In 2019, NHS Resolution (the body tasked with the unenviable job of settling NHS claims and disputes) estimated the total cost of all outstanding compensation claims to be £83 billion. Incredibly, this is nearly two thirds of NHS England's total budget for 2018/19 of £129 billion.[1]

Health services worldwide are not unaware of this major safety and cost issue. Here in the UK, there has been much media and regulatory discussion and debate about medical deaths and complications, with institutional NHS disasters like the Bristol baby scandal, *Mid-Staffs* and the Shrewsbury and Telford Trust, as well as rogue individuals like Shipman, Patterson and Allitt all driving much publicity, as well as new mandatory NHS and regulatory requirements for frontline healthcare staff to speak out in the event of witnessing or suspecting neglect, cruelty, mismanagement, inappropriate risk-taking or cover-ups.

Yet this is a position of the utmost hypocrisy, as my own experiences have clearly demonstrated. In UK healthcare in particular; providers, NHS executives, regulators and government ministers continue to publicly posture, spin, bleat and tweet about the mandatory duties of honesty, integrity, candour and speaking up that they have imposed upon front-line staff, whilst continuing, behind the scenes and in classic Orwellian *doublespeak*, to covertly oversee the truly brutal persecution, prosecution and destruction of whistle-blowers' careers, health and families in the endless and ruthless pursuit of NHS reputation management and organisational damage limitation.

As such, and particularly in the light of the most recent NHS scandals mentioned above, the fight for the absolute right to provide full, frank and honest disclosure without risking immediate career-ending retribution continues to be powerfully relevant to both public safety and public finances; as does the right to receive appropriate, fair and ongoing protection and treatment after such acts of social and professional safeguarding.

---

[1] https://www.bbc.co.uk/news/health-51180944.

WHISTLE IN THE WIND was written primarily to set the record straight and to rebut several serious attempts to misconvey events and misappropriate responsibility over my career destruction and dismissal from the NHS; these events coming shortly after speaking out about key safety failings to the Care Quality Commission (CQC).

After I'd been illegally dismissed from my post as consultant surgeon by the University Hospitals of Morecambe Bay NHS Foundation Trust (UHMBT) – my employer for 16 years, the entirely unfounded rumour was put about that I had hurriedly left under a financial cloud. Ex-colleagues and ex-patients were left with the clear, uncontested impression of some kind of financial impropriety, and a rushed resignation in disgrace. As events were to prove, this couldn't possibly have been further from the truth. Nevertheless, claims were made, even under oath and during the subsequent litigation, that I had claimed considerable sums of NHS monies to which I was potentially not entitled. Yet, as the 2018 employment tribunal was to unanimously confirm, it was the NHS itself who had been deliberately unlawful all along, knowingly withholding a substantial five-figure sum of my legitimate earnings and threatening to help themselves to a good deal more; whilst also knowing full well that it was in the wrong, fabricating counter-allegations against a whistleblower and clearly expecting, by corporate intimidation, *doublespeak* and legal *force-majeure* to get away with such illegality and wrongdoing.

Repeatedly subject to additional accusations of prejudice, poor standards, bullying and racism, it was, I believe, precisely the stance that I and others took on excluding such behaviours from our department and my absolute, unconditional refusal to bend and compromise on the NHS's Behavioural Standards Framework and professional ethics which clearly cost me, firstly, the joint departmental lead post and, entirely predictably and shortly afterwards, my entire NHS career and vocation itself.

There can be few things more destructive to someone's career than being formally and officially subject to revenge-accusations of prejudice, malpractice, financial irregularities and racism; particularly when such allegations are profoundly weaponised by the victim being unable to defend themselves or point out the wider context and retaliatory background to such vexatious counter-allegations. Indeed, in describing how it feels to be on the receiving end of such horrible and unfounded accusations – it is the career equivalent of unexpectedly having acid thrown in your face.

Immediately damaging; corrosive and blindingly painful, and in the case of any genuine whistleblower, entirely undeserved. But by far the worst is in the long run, as such actions leave a predictable, horrible and permanent career disfigurement and disability that can never, no matter how skillful the reconstructive surgery, be fully repaired or set right.

As an enduring, feral and intensely public marker of career-hate, it has very few equals.

Subsequently accused by the NHS of having no case; threatened and bullied with potentially devastating six-figure costs in the subsequent employment tribunal, with NHS executives and their solicitors aggressively asserting their confidence that I had no credible or winnable case in law, the reality couldn't possibly have been more different. In truth, my ex-employer had already accidentally but definitively revealed their employment law guilt, only to cynically have the hard proof of such NHS culpability struck out on a technicality as *inadmissible evidence* (see page 178 of *Whistle in the Wind*).

These tactics, and the others revealed later in this book, reduced what should have been a respectful, truthful judicial process of the highest standards to, in my opinion, a shallow, corrupt and disgraceful NHS funded legal farce.

UHMBT's current Chief Executive was quite right to state that, in hindsight, the case should never have been contested.

Yet, this is not how it works in the tainted, disorientating and Orwellian world into which the vulnerable, well-meaning, naive and solitary whistleblower stumbles. Over and over again, the organisation that has sanctioned or expelled the whistleblower proceeds to twist and distort reality; never admitting responsibility, but insistently seeking to impose a sanitised and censored, Alice-through-the-looking-glass corporate version of events upon the unprotected and usually lonely, confused, isolated and sometimes jobless whistle-blower. And all too often, as detailed in my first publication, the individual whistleblower at the heart of such a process, seeking simple legal redress for being illegally and hypocritically punished for nothing more than safeguarding, doing their job and discharging their public, social and professional duty, finds themselves instead falsely recast as the wrong-doer and sorcerer in an exercise of corporate gaslighting that has all the integrity of a medieval witch-hunt.

———————

UNFORTUNATELY, SINCE THE PUBLICATION of *Whistle in the Wind*, a new slew of allegations and 'evidence' has found its way on to the record. Some allegations have been ridiculed and disproven almost immediately. Some were truly ludicrous; comical even, right from the start. But others have found a frightening; indeed, terrifying degree of traction. Yet again, I find myself in the situation of either capitulating to the deny, degrade and destroy tactics of a state monopoly that seems ruthlessly intolerant of independently thinking employees with a social conscience, or wearily once more taking to self-publication to refute the latest manipulations, smears, falsifica-tions, investigatory distortions and newly fabricated allegations and, in the absence of any other attempt at an impartial account or investigation, give my side of the story.

With the publication of 2019, media attention, the end of the liti-gation process and the various statements made to press and regulators, this whole distressing episode should have ended two years ago. Lessons learned, apologies made, wrongs righted, honest facts published, responsibilities acknowledged and a determined effort made to avoid further cover-up, repetitions, retaliation and further spoliation of evidence.

But instead of drawing a candid and defining line under this whole sorry sequence of events, the converse has, in my opinion, happened; with *Whistle in the Wind* instead heralding a new round of NHS spin, smokescreens, gaslighting, prejudice and hate, and a truly dystopian, dogged determination to covertly rewrite the reality and crush, by whatever means possible, and perhaps most importantly be clearly seen to crush and silence the dissenting individual whistle-blower.

Just recently, and in a written response to my anxiety, disorientation and distress over the above tactics, tainted evidence and the ongoing damage to what very little was left of my self-esteem and clinical reputation, I was menacingly told...

...you wanted this from the outset Peter.

Except that I didn't. Far, far from it. All I wanted was for the truth to be told and the spin, cover-ups and risk-taking to cease.

In the context of such a coarse, threatening and intimidating statement and the events of the last two years, *Whistle in the Wind's* contribution to exposing wrongdoings and risk-taking, and its attempt to negate the systematic targeting of whistleblowers in UK healthcare is clearly far from complete.

IN SOME AREAS *Smoke and Mirrors* will overlap with its sister publication, for which I apologise, but there is plenty of new material and much that I could, and perhaps should, have predicted. This new manuscript will, I hope, help to further detail the pitfalls, resistance, smears and retaliation that await those public and private sector whistleblowers who put social, humanitarian and professional obligations ahead of career, comfort, convenience and the seductive attractions of a quieter, easier and more secure life.

My position on NHS standards, cover-ups and the regulatory oversight of the healthcare system remains entirely unchanged. Indeed, my opinions have hardened, and there is no point revisiting the issues dealt with in the introduction to *Whistle in the Wind.* However, my personal insights into organisational secrecy, local and national politics, regulatory bodies, evidential concealment, electronic manipulation and perjury have greatly expanded. I intend to work all of these into the narrative.

Please bear with me as I take you through another two years of intense personal, professional and family hell. It is not a pretty story; far, far from it, with issues that many will find upsetting and others will consider ugly, relentlessly negative and possibly even inappropriate for publication. Unlike *Whistle in the Wind*, where, on occasions, I attempted to lighten the reader's burden with some humour, there is very little that has come out of the last truly awful two years that is worth laughing about. However, it is only by telling these brutal and corrupt stories in their hideous fullness that we can perhaps embed within our healthcare system and wider society a determination to establish a fairer, kinder, safer and more honest culture for our friends, families, dependents and those who will follow us.

Whistle in the Wind was a relatively simple and clean story; a chronologically sequenced, depressingly well-trodden corporate death-dance of state sponsored vocational assassination, and a choreographed pathway of career destruction already well-beaten by those worthy NHS whistleblowers who preceded me.

Smoke and Mirrors, on the other hand, is of necessity much more fragmented and will appear, at first sight, to be significantly more disorganised. It will, I am afraid, be much more demanding and, rather than a consistent and relatively seamless chronological story, the narrative will take the reader off in a number of different directions. External investigations, General Medical Council (GMC) cross-examinations and further revenge-allegations, COVID, lockdowns and border closures, an increasing sense of homelessness and helplessness; secretive reports, psychological and evidential gaslighting, family separations together with various meetings and presentations are all intertwined. Please bear with me as I try and draw the last two years together into a coherent sequence.

Part I of the book will, in a roughly chronological order, bring the reader up to date with the events since the writing of *Whistle in the Wind*.

Part II is the story of the last seven years, as seen from the perspective of the bereaved family of *Patient A* from *Whistle in the Wind* – Mr Peter Read.

Part III serves as an updating and expansion of the points made in the postscript of *Whistle in the Wind,* and will attempt to elaborate upon, update and learn from the multitude of errors and omissions made by the NHS itself, the quangos and regulators who oversee our national standards, and, of course, the law.

Drier and almost certainly less compelling than Parts I and II, Part III is nevertheless a necessary part of the story. After all, the whole point of *Whistle in the Wind* was to provoke discussion and debate over the current NHS and wider societal whistleblower hypocrisies. And whilst it may not make such good storytelling, an overview of the legion of failures documented in these two publications is a necessary addendum if both books are to attempt to fulfil their intended purpose. To question, inform, stimulate both debate and constructive change and, perhaps above all, to play some small role in putting an end to the bullying, hypocrisy, fear, double standards and cover-up culture that seems to permeate every corner of our National Health Service and indeed our wider public life.

Once again and regrettably, the book will have to be self-edited. I hope the reader will allow for this, and excuse any lack of clarity as I try and make sense of all these variables (perhaps for myself as much as for the audience), untangle the different threads and present the ongoing story with as much evidential backup as possible. There are a number of repetitions in the text, particularly with respect to the events of December 2014. I sincerely apologise in advance for this, but have made the decision to leave these in for the simple reason that they emphasise certain points, let the story flow and allow the reader to avoid constantly having to check back to previous facts and statements. For those who are not familiar with the facts published in *Whistle in the Wind,* I will try and incorporate sufficient information to allow the reader to make sense of the events prior to 2019, hopefully without losing the attention of those more familiar with these events, or labouring and repeating points unnecessarily. I hope that the reader will forgive me in the event of the latter. I would sooner be criticised for repetition than for a lack of clarity, position or continuity.

For those who are unfamiliar with the discourse leading up to and after my constructive dismissal from UHMBT, or for those who wish to refresh their memory of these events, a timeline of the core events covered by *Whistle in the Wind* is also included at the end of the book.

WRITING ABOUT THIS ONGOING SEQUENCE of different, profoundly life-altering events and trying to explain it from the viewpoint of my entire family as well as close friends, colleagues, patients and relatives has not been at all easy. I'd hoped that setting it all down in the form of another book might give me some kind of deeper perception and understanding of recent events. Peace, comprehension and insight perhaps, instead of my overwhelming sense of bewilderment, confusion, fear, disbelief and injustice. However, even setting aside the potential traumas of publishing that lie ahead, revisiting the last two years has emphatically not been the cathartic exercise that I had hoped. Rather more, a loaded march through the modest highs and, mostly, extreme lows of sometimes terrifying emotions.

Brought up in that dubious British tradition of stiff-upper-lip, it has been incredibly difficult to write about the soul destroying extremes and intensity of the last two years. But emasculating the emotion would be like remastering HD video in grainy 1960's black and white. Indeed, in the feedback and learning from *Whistle in the Wind*, it is clear that it was the emotional rollercoaster of 2014 to 2018 which seemed to draw readers in most powerfully. I will therefore try to work the appropriate emotive and psychological narrative into the text, but without allowing it to become overbearing, self-pitying or excessive.

SMOKE AND MIRRORS was originally conceived as a response to the events of the last 24 months and, at least in part, as an answer to the external NHS England investigation into the UHMBT urology department. At the time of writing, the conclusions of this NHS funded private investigation have not yet been finalised. I have therefore deliberately delayed publication until after the investigation has concluded. Bearing in mind the media attention which these issues have received previously, I fully expect that the findings of the investigation will be widely published, potentially causing further serious and permanent damage to my reputation and career. Consequently, *Smoke and Mirrors* is my immediate response to this. I hope that this new book will be read alongside the conclusions of the investigation in order to give the full picture, set the record straight and clear my name.

With the NHS England investigation turning up new disclosures which purport to profoundly alter the facts and evidence portrayed in *Whistle in the Wind,* together with what appears, from my perspective, to be a dramatic and chilling change in the NHS's strategy towards myself and my family, I believe, as above, that it is overwhelmingly in the public interest for me to publish my own account of the last two years. There may well be further and potentially very serious personal repercussions and retaliation from ex-colleagues, the NHS and my medical regulator. However, above all else and regardless of the price that I pay, I will not, under any circumstances whatsoever, be silenced over fundamental issues of patient safety and organisational probity and integrity, irrespective of whether or not this costs me what little is left of my medical and surgical career, reputation and registration. As *Smoke and Mirrors* will clearly demonstrate, and as the ongoing Post Office *Horizon* software scandal has definitively proven, in this brave, new and overwhelmingly digital world, none of us can consider ourselves safe from electronic, evidential and psychological distortions and manipulation. And no one is more vulnerable to such tactics than the defenceless and detested whistleblower. Damned, discriminated against and displaced for doing nothing more than take an intensely lonely stand against a huge state monolith over risk-taking, dangerous practices, cover-ups and patient harms.

There is, I believe, a clear and overwhelming public and civic interest and indeed professional duty in publishing my latest account without delay.

IN THE CONTEXT OF PROFESSIONAL DUTY, regulatory requirements, candour, safeguarding and freedom to speak up, *Smoke and Mirrors* should be regarded in its entirely as another act of openness, candour, whistleblowing and social disclosure in itself. However, whilst *Whistle in the Wind* faithfully documented the well established, well-trodden pathway of corporate whistleblower retaliation, my more recent experiences have opened up a whole new vista of anti-whistleblower abuses. A chilling new panorama of backdating, psychological manipulation and gaslighting which came terrifyingly close to claiming another life, whilst simultaneously and permanently discrediting and closing down the safeguarding issues highlighted in *Whistle in the Wind* and burying them all....

Once and for all and forever.

This new publication is therefore a necessary professional responsibility and obligation in countering the *Smoke and Mirrors* of the last two years and is, as above, a further act of safeguarding and candour in itself.

Many readers will appreciate the intense irony of the fact that my ex-employer, the National Health Service, and my medical regulator, the General Medical Council have both laid on a very public and noisy display of virtue-signalling and support for whistleblowers in recent years, going so far as to make acts of candour, safeguarding and whistleblowing a non-negotiable requirement of employment and registration. Yet, in a truly textbook display of Orwellian *doublespeak* and hypocrisy, both have been at the very cutting edge of the latest retaliatory actions, harassment and prejudice that have been indelibly etched not only into my own life but also that of my family over the last decade.

Once again, patient names and the names of any third parties who are not immediately relevant will be concealed. Importantly, I have been legally advised to redact the names of those ex-colleagues who are subject to current GMC investigations. Accordingly, these ex-consultant colleagues are referenced as individuals A and B. Screenshots of emails have also been redacted, but where neutral third party email addresses have simply been erased, the redactions relating to my ex-colleagues are also overwritten with A or B. I apologise for the additional lack of clarity and readability that these legally necessary redactions bring to the book.

On this occasion I will not have a detailed witness statement or legal bundle to follow, but, as with *Whistle in the Wind*, the manuscript will follow the evidence in a roughly chronological sequence.

Like *Whistle in the Wind*, the book will be priced to recoup costs, rather than to make a profit. If I can achieve only a small fraction of the sales achieved by the previous publication then this alone will more than justify the effort and investment.

I remain deeply indebted to everyone who took the time to purchase or share a copy of *Whistle in the Wind* and review my story, especially to those who went to the effort and trouble to leave feedback, or who approached and supported me personally.

Thank you, all of you. Especially those of you who are ex-colleagues and friends from my previous life in UHMBT.

For those who wrote or emailed but did not receive a response from me – I can only sincerely apologise. Pressure of work, as well as travel home and recent non-urological commitments have dominated the last 24 months. I will try and do better this time....

I hope that my second publication will coherently build upon the first, and help to further inform the current debate and struggle over safeguarding, candour, public safety, state-sponsored retaliation and harassment, evidential tampering, investigatory powers, backdating, impartiality, spin, employment law and the relevance of a plethora of regulatory bodies; so many of which seem to serve little or no purpose other than projecting an image of order, fairness, public safety, lawfulness, oversight and regulation where, in fact, none actually exists.

Peter Duffy,
Lancaster,
24th December 2020.

Acknowledgements

ONCE AGAIN, MY FAMILY must take pride of place. Fiona, Edward, Robert and William have, I feel, been viciously punished for my candour and safeguarding every bit as much as I have. Already into our fifth year of separation, who could have guessed that in early 2020, a global pandemic would isolate us from each other even more brutally than before. Nevertheless, here we all are, just hours before Christmas 2020, together at last for a decent quality and quantity of home-time for only the second spell in the last year, something, in the midst of a terrible 12 months, that can be unequivocally celebrated. So far, we have, together, managed to endure, rather than fracture and capitulate.

Particular thanks to my wife Fiona for her ongoing support and tireless efforts in proof reading and correcting my typography and punctuation in this latest publication.

The family of Mr Peter Read (Patient A – the *avoidable death* case from *Whistle in the Wind*) Karen and Nicola Read have been simply wonderful. Where others might very reasonably have been hostile or resentful, they could not possibly have been more supportive. Never was their support more badly needed than during the weeks and months of extreme agony after new email allegations unexpectedly emerged (but more of this later).

My wider family have also, as always, been unswervingly supportive. My mother Jean, sisters Clare and Louise and brother Chris. And, of course, the influence and ethics of my father Francis, who sadly died in 2010 – but who most certainly lives on in my determination not to be silenced over these issues. We are, after all, a product, both biologically and morally, of the immediate family that we grow up with.

In that context of childhood and adolescent influence, my old friends Mike, David, Andrew and Mark have again been robust and unwavering in their support, even though I've seen them just the once over the last year.

Alison Birtle, Professor of Clinical Oncology and Colin Cutting, Consultant Urological Surgeon have shown considerable courage and have been consistently there for me in their desire to help to establish the truth. They have encouraged me to keep going where, so often, the temptation to give up was overwhelming. I am also grateful to the other UHMBT staff who have had the courage and integrity to keep in regular touch and support me. I dare not name you, for your own sakes, but you know who you are and I am most grateful.

The British Medical Association (BMA) have remained supportive, but this year it has been the Medical Protection Society (MPS) who came good. The BMA deal, amongst other things with employment law issues and I remain indebted to them for their assistance during the employment tribunal of 2018. This year has been defined by counter-allegations and counter-evidence of neglect and negligence, taking us deep behind the lines and into the hostile lands of GMC enquiries and private investigatory organisations. This is the territory of medical defence and indemnity organisations and the MPS came good, with the support of solicitor Ms Jane Lang and medico-legal adviser Dr Clare Devlin.

Protect (formerly *Public Concern at Work*) have encouraged me and remained in touch.

We are blessed with several quality MPs in the North West of England. Trudy Harrison, Conservative MP for Copeland in North Cumbria; Lord Walney (formerly John Woodcock, Labour MP for Barrow and Furness), Cat Smith (my own Labour MP for Lancaster and Fleetwood) and Tim Farron (Liberal Democrat MP for Westmorland and Lonsdale) all came together in a remarkable cross-party consensus to request a formal investigation by Matt Hancock, former Secretary of State for Health and NHS England. Lord Walney has recently stepped down, taking a seat in the House of Lords, and been replaced by Simon Fell, Conservative MP for Barrow and Furness.

They have all been extremely supportive and I am very very grateful to them all.

The staff of Noble's Hospital, Isle of Man have remained both a support and a true inspiration, particularly during the late winter, spring and summer months of 2020 as COVID-19 crossed the Irish Sea and seemed set to devastate the nursing and residential homes of the Island. All at once supportive and sympathetic, it has been a pleasure and a true and lasting privilege to work alongside them. Their commitment, humour and endurance in no small measure endowed me with the determination to do my own bit for the local population.

Nicola Thatcher, Consultant Solicitor has again been extremely generous of her time and has assisted me with a legal opinion on the text.

Thanks too, to my immediate colleagues at Noble's Hospital; Steve, Julie, Jackie, Emily, Marie, Claire and, more recently, Ade, Milan and Baher as well as my other surgical, nursing and medical colleagues.

And finally, my family again.

Surely, now – at last, things can only get better?

Contents

Foreword xix

Prologue xxi

Acknowledgements xxxiii

PART I: Unforgiven 1

CHAPTER ONE: Hostile Cross-Examination 3

CHAPTER TWO: Publication 13

CHAPTER THREE: Amy Fenton, MPs, and a Statement in the House ... 21

CHAPTER FOUR: The Fallout 27

CHAPTER FIVE: Retaliation by Referral, Yet Another GMC
Investigation 35

CHAPTER SIX: Board Meeting 51

CHAPTER SEVEN: Second RCA 55

CHAPTER EIGHT: The Independent Urology Investigation, Niche's
First Meeting 75

CHAPTER NINE: Anonymous Tip-off 77

CHAPTER TEN: Morbidity and Mortality Meeting 81

CHAPTER ELEVEN: Pandemic 87

CHAPTER TWELVE: New Evidence 101

CHAPTER THIRTEEN: Decision 123

CHAPTER FOURTEEN: Questions 125

CHAPTER FIFTEEN: AfPP 139

CHAPTER SIXTEEN: More Questions 143

CHAPTER SEVENTEEN: Proof 161

PART II: Peter Read's Family's Story, By Karen Read 179

**PART III: The rankest compound of villainous smell that
ever offended nostril** 197

INTRODUCTION: Legion of Failures.. 199

CHAPTER ONE: The NHS, Lessons Eternally Unlearned 205

CHAPTER TWO: The Regulators... 215

CHAPTER THREE: The Law 223

POSTSCRIPT: Cover-up and Carry-on.. 243

Epilogue.. 253

ADDENDUM: Déjà Vu 257

Timeline.. 262

Glossary 271

PART I

Unforgiven

CHAPTER ONE

Hostile Cross-Examination

THERE WASN'T ANY WARNING, simply a General Medical Council (GMC) email out of the blue, late on Tuesday afternoon, the 23rd April.

Spring 2019. The cathartic construction of *Whistle in the Wind* was pretty much complete but unpublished, and the traumas and horrors of the NHS's and Manchester Employment Tribunal's treatment of me had mostly receded from my consciousness, at least during busy working days. Night-times were a different matter, but at least I could work and, occasionally, play without constant flashbacks, palpitations and reminders of the whistleblowing, NHS retaliation and career fallout of recent years.

Now, in a split second, they were back. And with a whole new intensity.

The GMC oversees the medical profession's standards as well as individual doctor's registrations. By and large, most doctors regard them with fear rather than admiration. Whilst they are generally thought of as fairly rigorous, they tend to move at about the speed of the Lancaster Canal and produce verdicts against doctors that can, in my opinion, generally be classified into 'sound', 'unsound' and 'howler' categories (see Dr Bawa-Garba for an example of the latter). To be fair, the former category dominates.

Having previously expressed serious concerns about three NHS consultants (see *Whistle in the Wind*), The GMC had specifically questioned me about the clinical standards of one of those ex-colleagues – Mr Madhra, just a few days after my first 2018 employment tribunal hearing ended. Now, twelve months later, they requested that, as a part of their ongoing investigations into Mr Madhra's consultant conduct, I attend a hearing of the Medical Practitioner's Tribunal Service (MPTS), a part of the GMC, on the 13th May, 2019.

Mr Madhra has now indicated that he wants you to attend the hearing to answer some questions regarding his case. I apologise that this is such late notice. Mr Madhra has only recently provided his request for your attendance.

Please can you indicate if you can attend the hearing in Manchester on 13 May 2019? If this is not possible, can you indicate if you can attend the following day on 14 May 2019? If it is possible for you to attend, the GMC legal support team will arrange any travel and accommodation that is required.

Thankfully the 13th wasn't a Friday and, as arguing with the GMC is (like NHS whistleblowing), usually a poor career move, I warily agreed.

THE GMC FLEW ME OUT and back again in a single day. Departure from the Isle of Man's Ballasalla Airport was a red-eyed 7am, with the now regrettably defunct Flybe (*Flybe-Maybe* to regular Manx travellers).

Arriving at Manchester Airport about 40 minutes later, I got to the MPTS building at around 8.30am. Shown into a rather austere waiting room, I spent the next couple of hours twiddling my thumbs, thinking of how much this reminded me of the employment tribunal, jumping at the occasional extra ectopic heart beat and wondering what further medico-legal traps now awaited me.

My reflections went on for some while, not least about how I could have had a decent lie-in and caught a later flight; but eventually a rather harassed looking solicitor hurried in. Introducing himself as one of the GMC's legal opinions, he profusely apologised for the delay. Mr Madhra had lodged another complaint and objection to the process. Please would I be patient whilst the tribunal considered the protest and produced a written response?

Leaning closer, he confided…

I've no idea why he's called you. That's the trouble with doctors representing themselves. If I'd been advising him, I'd have made it clear that the best place for you would be a million miles away from here.…

I was finally called at about 11am. The delay had, at least, given me time to think through the likely questions and what answers I might provide. On the way in I registered several members of the public, seated at the back of the cavernous hearings room and, triggering another run of palpitations, I was informed that there was at least one journalist present.

Having been sworn in, I was invited to take a seat, with Mr Madhra to my left, the GMC's counsel and legal advisers to my right and the panel straight ahead of me. It all seemed depressingly *déjà vu*, the only real difference being that there was no Paras Gorasia (my barrister from *Whistle in the Wind*) to offer me support or to jump in and object to inappropriate questions and behaviour.

Steepling his fingers in the best legal attorney fashion, Mr Madhra began his interrogation, informing me that I had been called to give evidence and that he would now formally cross-examine me.

You may use the answers 'yes' or 'no' so we can get this over with quickly. Is that clear?

Now, I was on your interview panel in 2000 for your consultant job. I deeply regret appointing you. You have brought much disrepute, difficulty and division upon the urological surgery department.…

Thankfully the GMC's counsel was awake and quick to act as a Paras-proxy, pointing out that it wasn't reasonable to expect any witness to be restricted to two monosyllables. It was also pointed out that it wasn't myself on trial, although it certainly felt that way.

I managed to choke back the retort that we seemed to have forgotten the anglepoise and electrodes and we settled down to business.

Quoting from the UHMBT media statement issued by Dr David Walker, Medical Director in 2018, I was asked by Mr Madhra about my withdrawal of a significant number of claims against the Trust on the opening day of my tribunal hearing, and about the UHMBT statement that all of the cases that I had expressed concerns about had been fully investigated. The implication of this question, it seemed to me, was that I'd had a weak case to start with and had simply crumpled on the first day and lost my nerve.

Mindful of the journalists and members of the public present, I couldn't let that go past without correcting it.

It's factually accurate to say that I withdrew quite a lot of legal pleadings from the employment tribunal on that first day. However, the panel ultimately accepted that this was in response to the UHMBT legal team threatening me with costs of up to £108,000 if I didn't drop the case. It was, I felt at the time, tantamount to witness harassment and intimidation, but I felt compelled to reduce my case to try and protect myself and my family from a hugely punitive bill. Also, although it is true that the Trust claimed, in the statement, to have investigated all of the nearly thirty-odd cases that I was concerned about, in actual fact, I think they investigated only about eight of them....

We moved on to some of the historical clinical cases that had been discussed back in 2018 during my telephone evidence, with Mr Madhra listing a series of cases that I'd expressed concerns over.

Mr Duffy, would you take us through the years that these cases cover?

Going through the list, it was clear that all of the cases mentioned by Mr Madhra related to the early-to-mid-2000's, the implication being that these cases were all clearly historical and time-expired.

You've missed one, haven't you? The wrong-side kidney cancer case from, maybe...2014, where the non-cancerous kidney could easily have been removed?

Mr Madhra was keen to move swiftly on from this.

Mr Duffy, you have reported three doctors to the GMC. Is that right? Three doctors? All Asian doctors. Yes? Yet a white doctor caused much harm in Lancaster. He carried out a laparoscopic nephrectomy (minimally invasive kidney removal), *damaged the inferior vena cava* (the main vein at the back of the abdomen) *the duodenum and superior mesenteric artery* (upper bowel and part of its blood supply). *Yet you don't complain about him. What does that tell us? Why did you not make a complaint against him? Can you tell us why?*

Well, well. Here we were once more. Back, yet again, to the weaponising of ethnic diversity and personal characteristics. Who would have guessed that this thoroughly nasty issue would raise its ugly little head again?

Taking a deep breath, mindful of this allegation being made in front of at least one journalist, and mentally revisiting the response that I'd prepared in the waiting room, I stumbled out the reply that, in fact, I'd been involved in protected disclosures involving at least six hospital staff during my career. Three were BAME (Black, Asian and minority ethnic). Three were not. I countered that this made me nothing more than a diligent and professional member of the NHS and demonstrated that I was certainly not racist, being prejudiced only against lax, dangerous clinical behaviour. Furthermore, in relation to the nephrectomy case, I pointed out that the operation in question had, in fact, been carried out by one of the other ex-colleagues (Mr B) that I'd expressed concern about; not by the *white* colleague, as stated by Mr Madhra, who had simply taken over the procedure and done his best to resolve the problems once the damage had been done.

Silence....

No one jumped in, commented or volunteered their own opinions. The silence seemed like an invitation to fill the vacuum with some more information, so I continued:

Of course, that's not to say that I haven't seen or heard of prejudiced, abusive or discriminatory behaviour in the urology department. Quite the opposite....

7

Going on, I detailed some of the more prejudiced comments that had been made over the years and witnessed or reported back to me, covering offensive comments about religion, homelessness, gender, ethnicity, sexuality etc. Recalling that such comments had come from the very individuals who had accused me of racism, I drew attention to a particularly misogynistic, derogatory and racist comment allegedly made by Mr Madhra himself about *white women* and their suitability for casual sex but not marriage. Purportedly made a good number of years ago to a group including European heritage nursing staff and reported back to me as the then-clinical lead of the department; I made the point to the panel that the comment had caused significant hurt and that I'd consistently opposed such offensive remarks, no matter what the source, making a particular issue, whilst sharing the interim departmental lead job, of repeatedly emphasising and circulating the NHS's Behavioural Standards Framework.

No one objected to me getting this off my chest either, so I thought I might as well keep the momentum going.

I pointed out the fact that my application for both the interim and definitive departmental lead jobs back in 2015 and 2016 had made a major play on my opposition to prejudiced, bullying and offensive behaviour like this (*Whistle in the Wind,* page 120), concluding by making the point that I felt that, as much, if not more than anyone in the department, I had tried to make the department genuinely inclusive and to fight against and eliminate such inappropriate behaviours.

In my opinion and as a direct consequence of the stubborn stand that I'd taken on these issues, far from being the source of prejudice, smears and hate, I'd ended up being the recipient.

Offering to elaborate on these facts and bracing myself for an immediate, belligerent and indignant outpouring of denials, I was comprehensively sandbagged by the hesitation, dithering, bluster and clear absence of any powerful and overt denial from Mr Madhra.

Well…I don't need that. But I can't stop you…. I have no knowledge…ahh…it was never put in writing….

The shocking lack of any immediate, forceful and outright denial hung pungently in the air, akin to a bad smell that no one wants to acknowledge or admit to. Throats bobbed amidst a jumbled sea of expressions of incredulity from around the panel and advisers. Eventually, someone closed their mouth with a slight snap, and we all got a grip of reality again; the Chair intervening to reassure Mr Madhra that the panel was not being asked to make a determination on that comment.

I caught the eye of the GMC's legal counsel. He looked like he was having a little difficulty with his legal poker face.

The morning wore on with a series of further questions, each one announcing a fairly obvious medico-legal trap for me. I can't recall the exact sequence of questions, but we covered the possible consequences of my whistleblowing for the families of those colleagues that I'd spoken up about. We covered whether I had repeatedly contacted patients late at night and asked them to make complaints about colleagues; counter-allegations of bullying against myself and whether I had ever been investigated for such insinuations, together with whether I had been *dismissed* from the role of joint clinical lead by the Trust.

The judge continued to remind Mr Madhra that I was there purely as a witness and that the hearing and GMC processes shouldn't be used as an attempt to create a *double-jeopardy* situation and put me back on trial again. In the end, and after the crash course in hostile cross-examination that the NHS lawyers had bludgeoned me with a year earlier, it wasn't too difficult to dodge the more blatant medico-legal bear traps.

Thankfully, I was able to point out my historical concerns about the consequences of my whistleblowing for Mr Madhra's family. Expressed in correspondence to the then-Medical Director in the early 2000's, I'd clearly wavered and put off reporting my concerns about clinical standards for some three months, directly as a consequence of my (thankfully) clearly-documented anxieties about the potential fallout and adverse long-term consequences for Mr Madhra's family and dependents.

Yes, I'd contacted two patients in the early evening (once each, and not late at night), in order to establish the truth regarding concerns that they were being covertly and falsely blamed for colluding together and being the architects of their own post-surgical and potentially life-threatening complications. I agreed that I had indeed been forcibly demoted by the Trust from the role of joint clinical lead after taking a robust stand over offensive, bullying and prejudiced behaviour in the department and refusing to back down over that position. Finally, clarifying the situation regarding the counter-allegations of abusive and racist behaviour against myself, I pointed out that these had been made in very secretive UHMBT meetings without my knowledge. Not only had clandestine, untrue, defamatory and highly offensive allegations been made against me, but I understood that at least one secretive meeting, almost certainly more, had also been attended by one or more external advisers from, I had been told, either the British Association of Physicians of Indian Origin (BAPIO), the British Medical Association, or both.

So yes, there had indeed been such allegations, but not only had I been prevented from responding and defending myself, I'd been kept entirely in the dark about the very existence of such meetings and allegations until well after my dismissal from the Trust. Recalling the-then Medical Director's comments that the Trust had *never found anything actionable* in relation to these covert allegations, I pointed out to the GMC tribunal that it was, in my opinion, clearly no coincidence that within months of these accusations being formalised and secretly circulated to both Trust executives and non-executive directors, UHMBT had gone on to pick a series of contrived and entirely unnecessary employment disputes with me, resulting in my forced resignation and illegal dismissal from the NHS.

RETIRING FOR LUNCH, as with the employment tribunal, I was reminded by the judge that I was still in purdah and under oath and therefore unable to talk to anyone in case I compromised my evidence. Feeling sick, with my heart throwing off irregular ectopic beats and with no appetite, I walked a few dozen metres to one of Manchester's public squares, completed my notes on the events of the morning and sat in the sun, trying to relax in the early spring warmth and wondering what the afternoon would bring.

There were no further questions from Mr Madhra after lunch, so the judge and one of the lay panel members took the opportunity to question me.

Would it be fair to say that your evidence, under cross-examination by Mr Madhra, might have been affected or influenced by your previous correspondence and interactions with him?

It was a fair question from the judge and I hope that I answered it equally fairly and accurately, pointing out that, whilst it is hard not to be riled or provoked by difficult and unfair allegations, I had answered the questions as accurately and impartially as I could, motivated only by a desire to convey the truth and comply with my oath.

The other question came from, I think, the lay-panel member, and took us back to the fact that I had responded fairly vigorously to the cross-examination. The question related to my statements, taken by telephone roughly a year previously which had been considerably meeker and more uncontroversial.

Again, it was a fair comment and gave me an opportunity to expand on the situation I'd found myself in during the aftermath of the 2018 employment tribunal. I pointed out just how intimidated, terrified and disorientated I'd been twelve months earlier. Although the main tribunal hearing was over, the verdict hadn't been delivered and I'd no idea if I'd won or lost, and hence no idea if I was going to be subject to six-figure costs. Almost all my old close colleagues and work friends had rejected me or dropped out of contact, and I was very fearful of retaliatory allegations to the GMC about me, in response to my whistleblowing.

Now, a year on from that awful time, things seemed to have settled down. I'd had twelve months to try to adjust to the new reality and come to terms with these unpleasant facts of life, and hence was (very naively as it would turn out) now less fearful of further life changing consequences and fallout from my candour than I'd been a year earlier.

Thanking me for my cooperation, the judge closed the session and I gratefully rose and left the room for my flight back to the Isle of Man.[2]

Surely, I concluded stupidly, the worst must now be well behind me, and there'd be no further acts of revenge....

---

[2] After I'd left the tribunal, Mr Madhra was permitted to place a statement on the record about his cross-examination of me. He stated that after leaving India, he has lived in areas which were primarily Caucasian and that he had never had any problem with Caucasian people and that actually he liked them.

CHAPTER TWO

Publication

WHISTLE IN THE WIND was published on 24ᵗʰ July 2019, just days before we were due to fly out to Italy on our treasured annual family holiday and not long after my GMC cross-examination by Mr Madhra.

The text was largely complete by January 2019 and, without any editorial or publisher support, I'd been totally reliant on family and friends for advice and encouragement. Initially a scruffy mess of badly formatted, jumbled chapters, by perhaps Easter I'd managed to pull the potential book together into something that was hopefully both readable and informative. Now there was just the question of should it be published and, if so, how?

Conventional publication was the obvious way. This involves, at the very least getting a professional and experienced editor, an agent and a publisher. My suspicion was that the book was controversial enough that I'd get precisely none of these. A few tentative enquiries quickly ruled this out. Conventional publishers didn't want to come within a million light-years of me. Nevertheless, family and friends were clear that giving up shouldn't be an option and I finally settled on self-publication.

This would never have been possible a few years ago, but the stranglehold exerted by the traditional publishers over the book market has been broken and DIY print-on-demand paperbacks are now very much possible.

There are a number of ways of doing this, but Amazon is the dominant player in the global self-publishing book market. Self-publishing without editorial guidance or the support of an agent is daunting in the extreme, but there is a surprising amount of free advice online, and in the end, this seemed the logical, and probably only way to go.

A good number of people, interested in publishing their own whistleblowing stories, have approached me for advice on how I put together the text of *Whistle in the Wind* without paying a ghost author or using an editor. Sadly, I don't have any fantastic insights or advice that is not already available many times over on self-help publishing sites, although I'd certainly encourage any wronged whistleblowers to publish their accounts, with, of course, the appropriate legal advice.

Everyone is different. Some people work best to a formulaic approach, allocating maybe 250 to 500 words-per-evening, or perhaps 45 minutes of work before bed. For me, writing is very sporadic and not something to be forced. I'll go days without producing anything – and then have a sudden burst of energy, producing perhaps 1,500 words in an evening, or alternatively going back, revising and polishing several chapters in one sitting. Certainly, I have no gift for spontaneous, once-and-for-all writing and everything documented in *Whistle in the Wind* was revisited and revised at least half a dozen times.

A quiet place with adequate time and space is essential and I probably worked most efficiently in my rented flat at weekends, with nothing to disturb me all day, or in my weekend five to six hour-long trips home to Lancaster.

A rough structure and mental image of the book is vital, as is an idea of the size. *Whistle in the Wind* was roughly 75,000 words. This sounds like a lot, but when you break it down into chapter-sized chunks, it becomes much less daunting. A standard page of *Whistle in the Wind* probably contained about 300 words.

Know where you want to start, and where you want to finish. The typical reader will like a clear start and laying out of the facts; a logical sequence to events and an equally clean, clear finish, whether it be happy, sad or, as in my case, perhaps best described as sobering and educational.

Early on with *Whistle in the Wind*, I purchased a small pocket notepad that I could scribble ideas into. This came out of my realisation that, so often, I'd have a good idea or recollection of an important event whilst out walking, driving or even during nightmares and flashbacks. Invariably, I'd resolve to work them into the book only, by the time I'd found some spare time and fired up the laptop, to find myself unable to remember the idea that I'd been so taken by about just hours earlier. Nightmares were particularly difficult to capture. I'd wake up thrashing around, soaked in sweat and with my heart thundering along; terrifying images, events or emotions so unbelievably intense that they'd be right there, in the room with me. Yet, if I didn't shakily write them down, by the morning the memories, so graphic in the darkness, would have simply melted away into my subconscious. Later on, my smartphone notepad sufficed for this purpose.

It is also worth setting yourself up with a fast, lightweight laptop with at least four hours reliable battery life, so that you're not limited to evenings at home, but can take advantage of the odd lunch-break, train trip or, in my case, travel home at weekends on the *Ben My Chree* ferry.

Voice recognition software and a good headset can be a godsend. All too often, when I'm typing, I get half-way through a punchy paragraph and find that, stupidly and frustratingly, by the time I've laboriously typed out the first half, I've forgotten the end of it. Few things can be more disheartening, especially when you've just created a possible killer-description or phrase. This doesn't tend to happen with voice recognition, but the downside of voice-dictation is that you have to be ever alert to typos and misinterpretations, especially with the spelling of names and places.

A mixture of voice recognition and traditional typing was, in my hands, the most productive and, once the rough chapters were fleshed out, I was careful to share them with my family at an early stage.

Fiona, my very-long-suffering wife was, in particular, an invaluable sounding-board; pointing out errors, duplications and grammatical howlers. It's important to have someone to closely supervise your work if you cannot acquire an editor or ghost author. A grammatically fluent family member with an eye for detail, who is close enough to you to be candid and honest and who will not shirk from pointing out omissions and errors is invaluable in self-publication.

Book covers are extremely important. In the conventional bookshop, the spine and cover should be sufficiently colourful and attention-grabbing that it almost jumps off the shelf at you. Nowadays with on-line sales, it's the thumbnail images that grab the attention. As *Whistle in the Wind* moved closer towards possible publication, I decided that I wanted a vivid cover with a surgical theme, bright, eye-catching colours and a picture that naturally drew the eye towards it. I'd already decided on the title, but had no idea of how to go about designing a cover.

99designs of Australia came to my rescue. For a few hundred dollars, they put out my specification and arranged for dozens of potential book-covers to be emailed to me from a selection of graphic designers. Looking through them with Fiona and the boys and picking out the best features of them all, I worked with the designer of our favourite cover to come up with something that, I hoped, was clean and vibrant, and which would stand out from the dozens of other book thumbnail images, all clamouring for the purchaser's attention. As long as the cover is created in the correct format, it can then be very simply uploaded to the Amazon KDP self-publishing website.[3]

The next thing was the text. Whilst I'm reasonably competent at typing, trying to format everything myself was a disaster. Fiona and Edward had taken care of any grammatical howlers but, as the basic text of the book drew closer to completion, I despaired of getting everything properly sorted out, chapters correctly numbered and referenced, paragraphs inset uniformly, and so on…. It was clear that I'd either have to spend many dozens of frustrating hours trying to clean it up, formatting it and converting the book into unfamiliar

---

[3] Gregoire Saul, graphic designer of Daft Cat Studio in Kendal produced the cover design for *Smoke and Mirrors* to a similarly high standard and a remarkably low cost. *DaftCatStudio.co.uk*

eBook software for publication, or simply give up and hand the manuscript over to the specialists.

BB eBooks of Thailand were the experts that I turned to. Their results were nothing short of miraculous and, unbelievably, they had the whole book turned around within about three days; transformed from a literary dog's dinner into an orderly, beautifully formatted piece of work that I no longer felt ashamed of. And all for not much more than $100. Not only did I receive the manuscript in various electronic publishing formats, but it also came in perfect and professional PDF and Word formats too. Worth every cent and highly recommended.

Lastly, and far from least, there was the issue of the legal situation. Clearly, the book was controversial and *edgy*, not something that any conventional publisher would go near.

I'd done the personal due diligence on this, making sure that I was familiar with defamation law and being careful to stick to easily ascertained facts and the *legal bundle,* the roughly 3,500 pages of documents and evidence submitted to the 2018 employment tribunal. Of course, truth is an absolute defence against a defamation action, and I was very careful indeed to stick to what I knew to be the truth and what could be proven.

Surely, a number of readers commented, *things can't really have been as bad as you made them out to be?*

In reality, they were actually considerably worse. However, I was ruthless about striking out anything that I felt would be difficult to substantiate. Nevertheless, I still needed a top-level legal opinion before I dared publish.

Nicola Thatcher came well recommended.

Nicola works for Keystone Law and has acquired a well-earned reputation for vetting controversial publications. Knowing the background, she spent a good week going through the manuscript.

Thankfully, she suggested relatively few changes; perhaps 6 to 10 sentences throughout the book, but I was more than happy to settle the invoice. The overall content and thrust of the book remained unchanged, I already had plenty enough issues to have sleepless nights over, and Nicola's bill (very reasonable considering the number of hours that she put in) was again worth every penny.

I finished up with a legally vetted, professionally formatted print-on-demand softback, eBook and kindle manuscript with a photoshop quality, professional-looking cover, all for under £4,000.

It only remained to set up a free Amazon KDP account (very easy), drag, drop…

and wait with bated breath….

———————

THE FIRST 24 HOURS or so after publication were the ultimate anticlimax.

Whistle in the Wind sold precisely one copy. Of course, it was to my main editor-by-proxy and grammar corrector; Fiona Duffy.

Never mind, I'm just about into the top thirty million global Amazon bestsellers….

And then my luck turned. Amy Fenton, regional journalist for the North West Evening Mail had been following my story throughout. With local MP John Woodcock making a statement on the book's contents in the House of Commons at Prime Minister's question time (see chapter 3) and Amy emailing a copy of the book through to UHMBT headquarters for a formal comment, we all got more than we'd bargained for. Trust headquarters sent an email out to all staff, warning them about the publication of a controversial book and clearly implying that this publication should be avoided by all dutiful employees.

HISTORICAL ISSUES IN OUR UROLOGY SERVICE
23rd August 2019

Dear Colleagues,

I wanted to write out to you all following a series of very public releases in relation to historical issues in our Urology service last week – including in the local press, social media, the publication of a book and a statement by one of our local MPs in the House of Commons on Thursday.

We were notified 24 hours prior to these activities and you will have seen the initial statement I gave the night before the formal release....

I want to remind colleagues that over our most recent past, we've developed a culture which encourages people to raise concerns, and where we investigate those concerns, ensuring we put into practice any learning to continue to make our service safer. We will continue to promote that culture in our organisation.

That said, the release of the book and the subsequent contact we've had from colleagues, patients and the families of those patients identified has prompted further action....

It is really unfortunate that these issues we have been dealing with have now been presented to the public in this way. This isn't because of any concern with the issues being in the public domain – as this is the way we work as an organisation – but presented as a book, headlines in the local press and social media creates worry and anxiety for our patients, communities and our colleagues without the opportunity to explain what has been done over that period to ensure our services are safe. We will be working quickly on the actions highlighted above to try and address these worries as best we can.

I hope this gives a bit more clarity as to our initial response to the publication and the actions we are now taking. In the meantime can I ask you all to recognise that some of our colleagues and patients will be feeling incredibly worried following the events of last week and for us to be kind, considerate and supportive of each other as we work through this.

We will make further communication as and when necessary to ensure colleagues are kept up to date.

———————

WITHIN 24 HOURS OF UHMBT circulating their discomfort over publication, my sales had sky rocketed.

Sitting in the holiday heat of that south Italian summer in 2019, gazing across the olive groves to distant, shimmering, smoky mountains, listening to the birdsong and cicadas, surrounded by my much loved and much missed family and watching the sales rack up and the feedback start to accumulate from hundreds of miles away was yet another truly surreal experience. We all took huge strength from the social media messages and support that poured in from friends, family, ex-colleagues and patients. *Whistle in the Wind* was, at one point selling hundreds of copies per day and, incredibly, got as high as number 58 in the Amazon best sellers list. The sales for August 2019 alone, to my complete disbelief, came to nearly 4,000. It was undoubtedly one of the top moments of my life, seeing the book listed on the same Amazon page as best-sellers like *The Hungry Caterpillar* and *This is Going to Hurt*.

At last, it seemed, the truth was out and I'd found a way to get my message and version of events across.

Now, after my candour, we just had to await the backlash.

CHAPTER THREE

Amy Fenton, MPs, and a Statement in the House

EVEN AS WE WERE PACKING and setting off on that 2019 summer Italian holiday, events were accelerating at home too.

Despite the complete absence of backing from regulators, ministers and institutions, I'd had good and reliable support from several local MPs, all the way back to a meeting with Cat Smith, MP for Lancaster and Fleetwood in early 2017. It was Cat who had convinced me to take my concerns to the GMC, despite my very real (and, as it turned out, well-judged) fears of retaliatory allegations. Soon, Cat's support was supplemented by that of Tim Farron, MP for Westmorland and Lonsdale, who agreed to meet with me and talk through my concerns during a visit to London in late 2018.

In early 2019, as well as keeping in touch with Cat and Tim; John Woodcock, then-MP for Barrow and Furness now got involved. With local journalist Amy Fenton relentlessly pursuing the story too, and a slew of stories in the North West Evening Mail, the book's release in summer of 2019 prompted John Woodcock to go public, announcing the publication in the last Prime Minister's question time at Westminster before the summer recess of 2019.

It is right that these allegations are treated fairly and without prejudice to either side, but what is not right is the way that the Trust is seemingly not learning the lessons of transparency.

It is refusing Freedom of Information requests made by our brilliant local newspaper, which has led the way on this matter. We all owe a debt of thanks to Amy Fenton, a reporter who is just not taking no for an answer.

She is being told time and again that she cannot have information from the Trust. The Health Secretary must look at this, and I hope that he will come back to us when the House comes back in September.

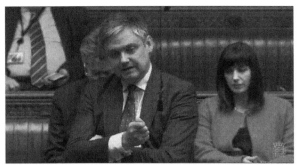

John Woodcock MP, 25th July 2019. House of Commons (Hansard)

John, Cat, Tim and Trudy Harrison, MP for Copeland all kept up the pressure on behalf of local constituents. Remarkably, considering that they represented pretty much the entire mainstream political spectrum, they all came together to write a powerful letter to the then Secretary of State for Health and Social Care, Matt Hancock.

HOUSE OF COMMONS
LONDON SW1A 0AA

The Rt Hon Matt Hancock MP
Secretary of State for Health and Social Care
Department of Health and Social Care
39 Victoria Street
London
SW1H 0EU

22 August 2019

Dear Mr Hancock,

**Re: request for formal inquiry into the
Morecambe Bay Health Trust urology department**

As MPs whose constituents are served by the University Hospitals Morecambe Bay NHS
Foundation Trust, we are writing to request that you order a formal investigation into
extensive allegations of failings in its urology department.

As John Woodcock noted in the House of Commons debate that preceded the summer recess
on 25 July 2019, Peter Duffy, a former consultant urologist at the trust who was effectively
constructively dismissed in 2016, has outlined appalling treatment of patients and severe
shortcomings in governance in a book, *Whistle in the Wind*, published last month. Mr Duffy
details the persistent mistakes of three of his consultant colleagues over the last 19 years and
the reluctance of the trust to address poor performance and protect him from seemingly
completely unfounded accusations of racism made anonymously when he tried to intervene.
Coroners have ruled mistakes were a factor in the death of two patients.

His book gives examples of how poor standards may have contributed to the suffering of
many others. As John said in his contribution to the debate last month, we urge you to study
this deeply alarming account which documents poor clinical and governance standards in the

trust over many years. Please also note that members of the public came forward to assert in our local newspaper, the Mail, that similar problems had resulted from substandard urology surgery.

As you may have seen, John's comments were echoed by Cat Smith MP, who said during the debate she saluted the work carried out by Mr Duffy and has asked your predecessor to take an interest in his case. Cat fully supports the call for a formal investigation into this issue.

Since then, only one of the three consultants responsible for the initial oversight has resigned and concerns remain of poor care in the department. Moreover, the trust has proved uncooperative in the face of these accusations and have attempted to obstruct an investigation into the matter by local newspaper reporter Amy Fenton, who has been working closely with Mr Duffy over the past year.

We would therefore request that you urgently consider commissioning a formal inquiry into the allegations of chronic poor practice and governance failings outlined in Mr Duffy's book. An inquiry could repeat the model followed by Dr Bill Kirkup, who was tasked by your predecessor in 2013 to examine failings in Furness General Hospital's maternity unit, following a number of neonatal deaths. The Morecambe Bay Investigation was sufficiently high profile, independent and transparent to instil public confidence without requiring the level of cost and process necessitated by a full public inquiry. Dr Kirkup, who previously distinguished himself as part of the Hillsborough Inquiry, examined specific failings and the management culture which allowed poor standards to persist and made a number of recommendations designed to improve transparency and patient safety locally and across the NHS, and ensure NHS whistleblowers are protected and valued. Published in March 2015, the findings of the Morecambe Bay Investigation were of great importance to your predecessor's focus on these issues.

The evidence provided by Mr Duffy strongly suggests the same trust is leaving patients at risk by failing fully to apply the changes which were universally accepted and promoted as a model for improvement by the department of health. We understand that you are likely to be d against launching an inquiry by managers of the trust who will point to action they have already taken, such as reviews they themselves have commissioned to address some of the problems outlined by Mr Duffy. We believe such existing steps are shown to be manifestly insufficient by:

I) the details in Mr Duffy's account, which describe the trust's reluctance to confront ongoing poor performance and failure to support Mr Duffy when he spoke out;
II) the members of the public now coming forward with fresh allegations, and
III) the obstructive and uncooperative attitude shown by the trust leadership towards both the whistleblower and the local media asking legitimate questions about the issues he and failed patients are raising.

It is also worth noting that before the Kirkup report was commissioned, the trust initially pointed to multiple internal and external reviews and scrutiny as evidence that any problems in Furness General's maternity unit were already fixed. Dr Kirkup showed comprehensively that this was not the case. We all have a responsibility to patients and to ourselves not to be falsely reassured this time.

We hope this persuades you to act to stop more urology patients being failed in Morecambe Bay and we are of course keen to meet to discuss the issue further. Due to the significant public interest in this matter we will be making this letter publicly available.

Yours sincerely,

John Woodcock MP
Cat Smith MP
Trudy Harrison MP
Tim Farron MP

At last, it seemed that there had been a genuine breakthrough, and maybe, just maybe, we were inching closer to proper, impartial scrutiny of exactly what had gone on, both in terms of clinical standards, cover-ups, contempt of the coroner's court, employment tribunal irregularities and clear breaches of the UHMBT board's promised protections for NHS whistleblowers.

Now that four powerful and influential local MPs were involved, representing the breadth of the political spectrum in the UK, surely there'd be no further corporate liberties taken with honesty and candour?

CHAPTER FOUR

The Fallout

RETURNING FROM SOUTHERN ITALY in late August 2019 was sobering in the extreme. As a family, we'd all fallen in love with the southern Italian way of life, surrounded by the beautiful, languid Italian landscape, centuries of history, architecture and art, beautiful food and wine and some of the friendliest and most charismatic people that we've been privileged to meet. Our villa was stunning and we'd cleaned out the pool and barbeque and packed our bags with real regret and, in my case, a sense of disquiet and foreboding.

I was quietly satisfied that I'd done the right thing and spoken out about the treatment dished out to myself, patients and colleagues, as well as the fear that so many NHS employees live in; the fear of being perceived as having spoken or acted out-of-turn and traitorously betrayed *The Organisation.*

I hoped that I'd got across the lose-lose situation that confronts a lot of NHS workers at some point in their lives when they witness dangerous or neglectful behaviour, as well as the difficulties in taking on a national leviathan and monolith like the NHS, together with regulators, Royal Colleges and guardians, all of whom, from my own experiences, would seem to have a vested and mutual interest in keeping things quiet and out of sight.

On the other hand, I was also more than a little overawed, indeed shocked at both the media response and at the sales figures for the book (already well over 4,000 sales – at least ten times my most optimistic hopes), but most of all, I hoped that by telling the truth, I hadn't landed myself and my family in yet another *double jeopardy* situation, where we'd all end up being tried, persecuted and possibly prosecuted all over again for the same *crime....*

Surely not? Not now that the local media and MPs had taken such a powerful stand on these issues?
Oh well, time will tell....

As late summer eased into a chilly and misty Autumn, the immediate media interest started to wane. Interviews with the BBC, Five Live, Radio Lancashire and the Lancaster Guardian came and went; but the attention span of the media is understandably short and the steady flow of articles that appeared over summer began to ebb away. However, behind the scenes, things were still moving.

In around September of 2019 and with the book still selling well beyond expectations, I received a rather unexpected invitation to visit UHMBT's headquarters at the Westmorland General Hospital for a face-to-face meeting with Aaron Cummins, Chief Executive of the Trust.

I'd never met Aaron before. He'd been high up in the Trust's executive during the death-throes of my career and vocation in 2016. However, it was Jackie Daniel (now Dame Jackie Daniel) who had presided as Chief Executive over my illegal dismissal that year. She had swiftly moved on, along with the then-chair of UHMBT, Pearce Butler in the weeks before my employment tribunal in May 2018. Dame Jackie had switched to Newcastle upon Tyne Hospitals NHS Foundation Trust and Pearce Butler to Blackpool Teaching Hospital NHS Trust. It was therefore left to Aaron to follow on and try and clear up the mess.

Never the sort of person to relish difficult conversations, I took some persuading before I agreed to go.

Walking back into UHMBT Trust Headquarters at the Westmorland General Hospital was bizarre and very unsettling. In many ways, it was just like I'd never left, with nods, smiles, handshakes, hugs and congratulations from a good number of clinical staff on the way in. Everything was just how I remembered it. However, the atmosphere in Trust headquarters itself was noticeably icier. The body language from several executives; stiff politeness together with gritted teeth, barely concealed behind rictus-like smiles left me in little doubt that I'd caused significant problems with my candour, and I'd not be forgiven for it any time this side of the next ice-age.

To be fair, Aaron was either not in this category; or perhaps he was better at covering up his emotions. Either way, ushering me into his office, we spoke candidly for some 45 minutes, covering many of the aspects of NHS whistleblowing and my own experiences. Aaron listened intently as I put forward my own impressions as to why the NHS and other big corporate entities seem congenitally incapable of welcoming candour and whistleblowing, instead seeming to treat any act of speaking out and safeguarding as though it were an unforgivable personal slight and act of extreme betrayal and treachery. Touching on whether I'd be prepared to take my old job back, I pointed out that it had been filled with indecent and conspicuous haste anyway, being advertised long before I left UHMBT and a new appointment being made just a few months after my dismissal. There was, therefore, no job for me to go back to anyhow. And also, whilst I genuinely believed Aaron's regret and wish to see me reunited with my vocation and family, it was clear to me that there were plenty of others in the organisation, and probably neighbouring NHS organisations too, who would be anything but welcoming.

It would be, I later observed to Amy, like being savaged by a wild animal, and then going back and sticking your head in its mouth again.

Nevertheless, I appreciated the offer. Aaron was persistent and persuasive but, as events were to show over the next 18 months, my decision to decline the offer and return to Noble's Hospital and the Isle of Man was undoubtedly the soundest decision that I made that Autumn of 2019.

———————

AROUND THIS TIME, I was also contacted by some of the ex-governors of UHMBT. Holding their posts during the period of the UHMBT midwifery scandal and the immediate aftermath, there was clear dismay amongst their ranks over another possible scandal. Despite all the assurances offered to them a few years earlier by UHMBT's executives and non-executive directors, and despite all the platitudes to the media about learning lessons, candour and a new era of openness and safety, it seemed that precisely the same issues that had triggered the midwifery investigation and the Morecambe Bay Kirkup report of 2015 had arisen all over again.

Most worrying to the ex-governors were issues relating to the Trust's treatment of whistleblowers. Several had already been involved in Sue Allison's whistleblower issues over breast screening, as well as the attempts that had been made in around 2012 to gloss over safety issues in the midwifery department. There was disbelief in the ranks of the ex-governors that more failings, including more avoidable deaths had been papered over, my own expressions of concern ignored and a coroner's order disobeyed; all of this being known to the UHMBT medical hierarchy even whilst the Trust was still proclaiming that they had learned and changed for the better, just months after the Kirkup report into the midwifery scandal had been published.

Even worse, and entirely unknown to me at the time, precisely these same issues seemed to be going on in parallel within the orthopaedic department at the Royal Lancaster Infirmary. Once again, these had been happening during precisely the period in which the Trust was busy assuring the media that lessons had been learned and the midwifery mistakes would never happen again. Yet, just as in urological surgery, it was alleged that errors and avoidable deaths had seemingly happened, with more unorthodox practices and counter-allegations against the whistleblowers. There was a rumour that an orthopaedic clinical lead had attempted to address these issues, yet had been forced to step down and move hospitals amongst counter-allegations of bullying and racism and, once again, a sense of the medical hierarchy and executives closing ranks to try and avert any scandal, whilst determinedly looking the other way over lapses in standards.

Only in the first few months of 2021 have these latest issues final-ly become public, but they were clearly known to the UHMBT board and executives years ago, and had also been causing considerable concern to the ex-governors for a good while, despite corporate reassurances.

Small wonder, then, that in late 2019, the ex-governors were troubled and, with the publications and news articles over the summer, it is greatly to their credit that, despite having stepped down and relinquished their responsibilities, a good number of them nevertheless remained engaged and committed to the local NHS service. Dave Wilton, Roger Titcombe, George Butler, John Pearson, Les Hall and Val Richards deserve particular respect in this regard.

With pressure from the local MPs, ex-governors joining in and an extraordinary council of governors meeting, there was building momentum for a full, external and independent enquiry to be commissioned. After discussions involving NHS England and NHS Improvement, a decision was made that a firm of private health investigators should be brought in by NHS England to undertake an independent and impartial investigation and look more deeply into the issues raised by *Whistle in the Wind*.

Niche Health and Social Care Consulting Ltd were ultimately chosen for the task and the contract announced in late November 2019, triggering a flurry of personal messages which arrived by letter and phone, my Noble's Hospital address, *Twitter* and *Facebook*.

I was roundly warned by a number of callers and letter writers to be extremely wary of any private investigatory firm employed and remunerated by the very same monopoly employer that I'd blown the whistle on, and the NHS Trust which had already behaved so abysmally during and after my dismissal. It was powerfully pointed out to me that the NHS had previously tried and failed to gag and break me with the aforementioned allegations of financial improprie-ty, prejudice, racism and bullying, as well as threats of life changing costs – and had probably spent well into six figures of public NHS funds in doing so.

This latest enquiry would, I was warned, simply be seized upon as another taxpayer-funded opportunity for the NHS to bring in what amounted to private detectives in an exercise whose ultimate aim, whatever the official line, would be to garner sufficient evidence to discredit me and close the whistleblowing issues down, by fair means or foul. Simultaneously, I was warned, the whole process would likely be spun as an *independent* enquiry, whilst actually creating an additional *double jeopardy* situation where I'd end up being put on trial yet again for the same *offences.*

However, to offset a number of worrying warnings, other messages portrayed Niche as tough, but also perfectly fair and reasonable and, as it is human nature to remember and nurse a grudge against things that don't go your way, I didn't pay too much attention to the more extreme cautions. After all, we all tend to move on from things that have gone smoothly, but to brood over and allow things to fester where we perhaps feel an injustice.

There was little to find out when researching Niche's background online and ultimately, it seemed that I'd simply have to form my own opinions as we went along.

The Read family were equally active in late 2019, pushing UHMBT repeatedly over the fact that they themselves had witnessed HM coroner, Ms Hammond, give a direct order that Peter Read's case (Patient A from *Whistle in the Wind*) should be discussed in the urology departmental Morbidity and Mortality (M&M) meeting. Five years on from that crystal clear court order, this still hadn't happened. Additionally, pointing out their dissatisfaction with the original UHMBT RCA (Root Cause Analysis) report into Mr Read's death from 2015 (which, of course, HM coroner had rejected later that same year), the family finally persuaded the Trust to concede that it would commission a fresh RCA. Negotiations over this began in late 2019, just as the news about Niche Consulting being appointed was published.

At last, as we moved towards the winter and the exit from 2019, heading for a new and, hopefully better year, we seemed to have some kind of momentum towards getting to the truth, with pledges about a proper RCA that would start again *from scratch* and an independent investigator who, I was assured, would be at pains to fearlessly follow the truth and the hard evidence, no matter where it led and without regard to their employer's well known historical antipathy towards whistleblowers.

2020.... A new year and new decade that I looked forward to with huge hope.

At last. And after all, as a family, we were well overdue for a really good year and a good few weeks of some quality time together....

What could possibly go wrong?

I'm sitting in the sun, my back against a warm brick wall. It's getting towards the end of our Italian holiday. The weather is bright and the clouds high and dazzling. Around me are creepers and climbing plants, resonant with flowers and greenery. The heat draws prickles of sweat from my forehead and, on the other side of the villa, I can hear the boys and Fiona; splashing, laughing and enjoying the coolness and relief of the pool.

On the patio next to me, two beautiful fluffy kittens are playing with a stray leaf, tumbling and rolling in the sunshine.

I watch them frolicking with carefree happiness. All is well, and it's lovely to see new life and innocence at play.

But as I watch, I suddenly sense that their playfulness is taking them nearer and nearer to a drain opening. Rolling over and over in their innocent games, all at once they're on the edge of the open drain. I lunge frantically to try and stop the inevitable – the awful knowledge already in my mind that I'm not going to be quick enough.

In slow motion, both kittens topple into the drain. I'm too late by a split second. Their pleading eyes look into mine as they slide into the foetid and stinking darkness.

And instantly, I'm pressed up against the open drain myself, head and one shoulder forced into the opening and my arm desperately reaching down, frantically groping and casting around, but neither kitten is within reach.

My eyes adjust to the stinking darkness. In the gloom I see one kitten carried away into the rank and filthy waters. It disappears from sight, mewing hopelessly. But maybe I can still save the second one. With a frantic lunge I force my head and shoulder deeper into the drain, the rough clay edges cutting painfully into my flesh. I grasp the second little kitten's sodden and stinking tail but, to my horror and panic, the last kitten begins to slip through my frantic grasp. Sliding head first into the reeking mire, she too is carried away out of sight, and I'm left struggling....

Gasping and fighting with the bedclothes and pillows and I realise that now, *I can't pull myself out and I'm suffocating; the stench is drawing me down, I can't breathe and I'm falling too...* and then I'm fully awake and thank God it was all just a dream.

I hope I didn't wake the lady in the flat below.

2am.

There'll be no more sleep tonight.

CHAPTER FIVE

Retaliation by Referral
Yet Another GMC Investigation

DISCLAIMER:

I've agonised long and hard over whether to include this chapter. It is deeply hurtful and I am aware that this plethora of defamatory revenge-allegations was sent through the internal UHMBT email system to at least one third party consultant, friend and ex-colleague; quite possibly a good number more. I can't even start to imagine the damage that these further behind-my-back allegations have done.

Counter-allegations to a regulator are a consistent and constant feature of medical and nursing whistleblowing cases (as in the GMC hearing of spring 2019), and, in order to complete my account, once again set the record straight and refute these allegations, I have reluctantly taken the decision to include this chapter.

2019 HAD BEEN A very eventful year and, other than the UHMBT board meeting, detailed in the next chapter, and correspondence regarding a fresh Root Cause Analysis (RCA) meeting (heading towards us early in the New Year) I'd hoped for a smooth and uneventful run into Christmas, New Year, the end of 2019 and better decade for both myself and the family. But there was still one more nasty surprise to come.

Thu, 14 Nov 2019

Dear Dr Duffy

I write to clarify that I have your correct email address in order that I may send you correspondence relating to a GMC matter. I would be most grateful if you could provide me with confirmation that this is your correct email address.

If this email address is not for the named addressee, please also confirm the same.

Thank you very much for your assistance.

Yours sincerely
█████ *Investigation Officer*
General Medical Council 3 Hardman Street, Manchester M3 3AW

It was a short and polite enough message, but I confirmed my details with a sense of foreboding. I'd been fully expecting some kind of revenge-referral ever since the GMC hearing in late spring and the publication of *Whistle in the Wind* in the summer, reckoning that any such referral would, after the initial correspondence and inquiries, probably land towards the end of the year. And here was the GMC, in November, double checking that they'd got my address correct.

Oh dear...I had a horrid feeling that I knew exactly what was heading my way....

In fact, the revenge-reporting of whistleblowers to their regulatory body is predictable enough to almost form part of the standard and routine process whereby individuals and organisations inflict their revenge on the whistleblower. I'd talked this through with Cat Smith, MP for Lancaster in 2017 and had pointed out to her that it was the fear of revenge allegations that had put me off going to the GMC well before the events of 2014 to 2016.

Such revenge-allegations against whistleblowers are predictable, regular and routine enough that the GMC even commissioned an investigation into the issue back in 2015.

Submitted under the title *The handling by the General Medical Council of cases involving whistleblowers. Report by the Right Honourable Sir Anthony Hooper to the General Medical Council*, it was presented in

March 2015, not long after Peter Read's avoidable death, and underlined the dilemma facing so many NHS frontline workers.

The report by Sir Anthony opened by quoting from the GMC's core publication 'Good Medical Practice' – essentially the core standards and behaviours that registered doctors are obliged to obey.

Paragraphs 24 and 25. Respond to risks to safety:

You must promote and encourage a culture that allows all staff to raise concerns openly and safely.

You must take prompt action if you think that patient safety, dignity or comfort is or may be seriously compromised.

a. If a patient is not receiving basic care to meet their needs, you must immediately tell someone who is in a position to act straight away.

b. If patients are at risk because of inadequate premises, equipment or other resources, policies or systems, you should put the matter right if that is possible. You must raise your concern in line with our guidance and your workplace policy. You should also make a record of the steps you have taken.

c. If you have concerns that a colleague may not be fit to practise and may be putting patients at risk, you must ask for advice from a colleague, your defence body or us. If you are still concerned you must report this, in line with our guidance and your workplace policy, and make a record of the steps you have taken.

Failure to comply with paragraphs 24 or 25 may amount to 'misconduct' and a finding that a doctor's fitness to practise is impaired. 'Good Medical Practice' states in paragraph 6 that: 'Serious or persistent failure to follow this guidance will put your registration at risk'.

So, no doubt whatsoever about the potential career-ending GMC sanctions that might be imposed on any doctor ignoring their mandatory duties of whistleblowing, candour, safeguarding, care and concern.

Having established the overriding duty, professional requirement and GMC enforced obligations of a doctor to speak out where there are patient-safety-related issues, Sir Anthony's report went on to state:

> The awful reality that emerged from Mid-Staffs and indeed other inquiries was that doctors knew about our guidance but were not empowered by it. They felt it was acceptable to 'walk by the other side of the ward' knowing that there was unsafe and unacceptable practice going on. We must all do what we can to make sure that does not happen again.
>
> There is considerable evidence that, in the workplace, persons who raise concerns about a danger, risk, malpractice or wrongdoing that affects others, may well suffer, or believe that they will suffer, reprisals at the hands of an employer or fellow workers.
>
> Employers and fellow workers may resort to reprisals against those who raise concerns in order to protect the reputation of the organisation or of a fellow (often senior) worker.
>
> Persuasive evidence that healthcare professionals who raise concerns risk reprisal and fear the risk of reprisal is to be found in the Submission by Patients First to The Freedom to Speak Up review.

Sir Anthony went on to quote directly from the Freedom to Speak Up review.

> In the introduction…Sir Robert (Francis) paints a bleak picture:
>
> The number of people who wrote to the Review who reported victimisation or fear of speaking up has no place in a well-run, humane and patient centred service. In our Trust survey, over 30% of those who raised a concern felt unsafe afterwards….
>
> This is unacceptable. Each time someone is deterred from speaking up, an opportunity to improve patient safety is missed.
>
> The effect of the experiences has in some cases been truly shocking. We heard all too frequently of jobs being lost, but also of serious psychological damage, even to the extent of suicidal depression. In some, sad, cases, it is clear that the toll of continual battles has been to consume lives and cause dedicated people to behave out of character. Just as patients whose complaints are ignored can become

mistrustful...staff who have been badly treated can become isolated, and disadvantaged in their ability to obtain appropriate alternative employment.

In short, lives can be ruined by poor handling of staff who have raised concerns.

The effect of the reprisals on individuals...is likely to be devastating. Doctors who have devoted their lives to the care of others face the prospect of their careers being brought to an end. One of the consequences may be that the doctor against whom the retaliatory measures are being taken becomes clinically depressed....

Sir Anthony concluded his investigation by stating:

In the context of this review, my concern is that employers may use the process of making an allegation to the GMC about a doctor's fitness to practise as an act of retaliation against a doctor because he or she has raised concerns or, simply, as an inappropriate alternative to dealing with the matter in-house.

If that happens, the GMC unwittingly becomes the instrument of the employer in its campaign against the doctor...the damage to the doctor can be lifelong.

...it would be both cruel and counterproductive to require doctors to speak up and then unfairly or inappropriately damage or destroy their careers when they do so.

...it must not be overlooked that any interference with or deprivation of a doctor's career has all the hallmarks and effects of harsh punishment for the individual and his or her family.

In a written submission to me, a senior legal officer in the GMC wrote: 'a medical practitioner can properly be criticised for not raising a concern, particularly where not doing so may compromise patient safety, even if doing so may lead to their being referred by their employer to the GMC for investigation and where the appropriate exercise by the GMC of its powers, including its powers to seek the imposition of interim orders, may have an adverse impact upon them'.

Sir Anthony closed his review by stating...

Whilst this may be right in law, doctors are not likely to raise concerns if they do not believe that they will be treated fairly by the GMC should an employer refer their fitness to practise to the GMC as a result of raising those concerns.

SURE ENOUGH, bang on cue and just as Sir Anthony Hooper might have precisely predicted five years earlier, barely had I informed the GMC of my correct details than a barrage of emails and allegations began arriving. The complaints against me, I was informed, were voluminous enough to be too big for a single email and, within minutes, nearly 30Mb of allegations were clogging up my inbox.

The GMC formally notified me of allegations:

- *That you have allegedly been racist towards Asian colleagues, bullied and harassed them and refused Asian consultants to take annual leave.*
- *That you have allegedly worked in a private capacity whilst on sick leave from the NHS.*
- *You allegedly failed to attend departmental meetings.*
- *You were allegedly dishonest regarding the availability of an on-call consultant including falsification of medical notes.*
- *That you have deliberately spoken about Asian colleagues in the media and asked patients to provide statements to the media.*
- *That you have published a book which is allegedly misleading.*

Going into the detail of the allegations had me sitting with my head in my hands, not knowing whether to laugh, cry or noisily break something.

Naming both the UHMBT Chief Executive and Responsible Officer in what appeared to imply corporate approval of my referral to the GMC, I had, seemingly *fallen very much below the expected standards over the past several years* and had *shown no improvements despite several actions being taken.* Having been *dismissed by the Trust due to his* (my) *unacceptable behaviour,* I was now *seeking revenge from the Trust.* I had, apparently, breached appropriate standards by publishing my *autobiography* which, it was alleged, I was distributing free as well.

It was furthermore alleged that my concerns had been *investigated thoroughly by the Trust, coroner, Royal College of Surgeon team, CQC and GMC and no cause for concern was found.*

The allegations went on...

and on...

and on....

In addition to being involved with financial irregularities while in this Trust, and his attitude and behaviour against the Asians and the Trust, he was also caught red handed working at the BMI hospital Lancaster while on sick leave.

He did not allow Asian consultants to take annual leave and his wife used to decide who gets what in his house in a Pizza party which he used to organise. He used to finger point and shout at the Asian consultants in front of the patients.

He is destroying the secular and democratic fabric of this country by saying that English consultants are superior in knowledge and skills as compared to people coming from Asia.

He is destroying the ethics of the NHS and teaching people new ways of bullying others. I am sure GMC will set an example by taking strictest possible action against him.

Lot of members of public are also condemning his un-called for behaviour.

Patient Mr ▇ *told us that Mr Peter Duffy rang him at night while he was asleep to tell him that ...(consultant A) has provided him with a wrong treatment.*

Furthermore, I was accused of taking all the bank holiday leave dates preferentially, confessing to taking intravenous crack and amphetamines at work, always finding some personal activity to do while on-call and asking for unusual favours from colleagues, who had to oblige, *otherwise he could be very aggressive and revengeful.*

One email from my ex-colleague accuser was signed off with the flourish – *it is the repeated nature of his behaviour which is worrying because other consultants who work in the same department are much better than him.*

I SHOULD HAVE BEEN DEEPLY SHAKEN at this latest development and knowing that these defamatory allegations had been covertly circulated within UHMBT's internal email system certainly caused me very considerable pain. However, as above, manipulating and exploiting the GMC's reporting procedures to ratchet up the pressure on NHS whistleblowers isn't exactly a new tactic, so, in the end, I acknowledged this new investigation with a sense of weariness, fatigue and resignation.

However, whilst not being particularly shocked at this tactic I was astounded to find, enclosed within the many hundreds of pages of allegations, a whole new slew of emails relating to my time in UHMBT and which I'd been entirely unaware of....

IN EARLY 2018 and in the run-in to the first tribunal hearing, I'd specifically asked again and again for disclosure of all internal correspondence, explicitly to include any allegations against myself and against others in the department from my consultant colleagues, Mr A, Mr B and Mr Madhra, and particularly with reference to counter-allegations of racism and bullying. With UHMBT seemingly equally determined to withhold such evidence from scrutiny, in the end, we'd been forced to go to a preliminary hearing and a judge's order to get any meaningful disclosure, as is required by law. Finally, just weeks before the first tribunal hearing began, we received the minutes of the covert departmental meeting from December 2014 (see *Whistle in the Wind* page 82) and the anonymous note to the police (see below) which had been sent within days of the covert meeting.

Lancaster Police
Marton St
Lancaster

Dear sir

I am writing to you to ask you to investigate Mr Peter Duffy consultant urologist of Morecambe Bay University NHS Trust for racism. Mr Duffy has caused much difficulty for consultants in department of urology. He has made unfair allegations /statements and has got other consultants in to trouble. I have complained to Trust but they take no notice. He has caused one consultant suspension and is making trouble for others. He is racist and makes other consultants feel isolated and in fear. He does not work hard and has favourable job plan but he complains about others and gets them into trouble. He is dangerous doctor and does not obey departmental head.

Mr PD is worthy of investigation by you for racism. All minority doctors in dept have suffered anxiety and stress and need to be interviewed by you. Do not ask Trust to investigate as PD seems to have extra immunity from Trust. Hope you will not show this letter to Trust but just investigate.

Sincerely yours

I, the judge, my legal team and the rest of the panel had been categorically assured, in the run-in to the tribunal and in a sworn statement from UHMBT, that there was no other meaningful and relevant internal correspondence to be declared in relation to these kinds of allegations other than some bland and directionless internal management emails regarding the anonymous police note.

Yet what was this? My ex-colleague's voluminous allegations to the GMC contained, explosively, a whole batch of previously undisclosed emails which had clearly been concealed from scrutiny by the tribunal, yet which UHMBT had clearly been under a legal obligation to provide and which had been requested again and again under the Data Protection Act and the civil laws on evidential disclosure.

Titled – *harassment, discrimination, unequal opportunities and abuse of medical governance against overseas consultants in Urology Department,* the emails, never seen before by either myself or the employment tribunal, clearly referred to the internal report of the meeting in which I was named as a racist, and gave a sense of the extent of the covert campaign of retaliation that had been waged against me in late 2014 and early 2015, at the same time that the anonymous allegations had been received by the police.

The redacted emails featuring the names of consultants A and B are marked as such.

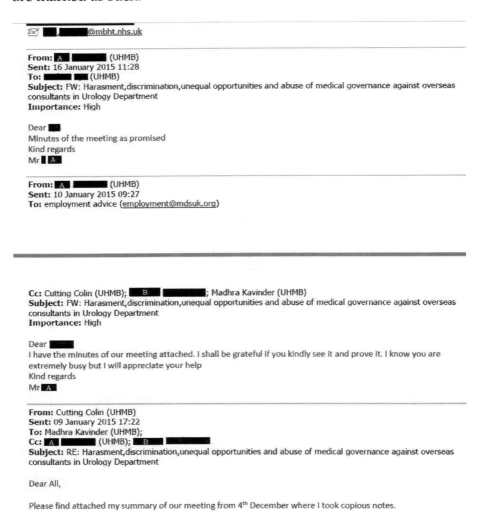

From: Madhra Kavinder (UHMB)
Sent: 07 January 2015 15:52
To: ███████ (UHMB)
Cc: Cutting Colin (UHMB); ▓A▓ ███████ (UHMB); ▓B▓ ███████
Subject: RE: Harasment,discrimination,unequal opportunities and abuse of medical governance against overseas consultants in Urology Department

Dear ███
I have not heard anything from you.
Could you kindly send me the minutes as I need to discuss this with non-executive directors.
kavinder

From: Madhra Kavinder (UHMB)
Sent: 31 December 2014 09:35
To: ███████ (UHMB)
Cc: Cutting Colin (UHMB); ▓A▓ ███████ (UHMB); ▓B▓ ███████

Subject: Harasment,discrimination,unequal opportunities and abuse of medical governance against overseas consultants in Urology Department

Dear ███
I refer to the meeting on 04-12-14 which was attended by myself ,Mr Cutting, Mr ▓B▓, Mr ▓A▓ and his union rep. and chaired by yourself.
1 Could I have copy of the minutes of the meeting please.
2 Could you please also let me know about the progress of steps take so far about the action plan made at the end of the meeting.
Mr K Madhra

From: ▓A▓ ███████ (UHMB) <███████.██@mbht.nhs.uk>
Sent: 13 November 2019 17:40
To: ███████
Subject: FW: Harasment,discrimination,unequal opportunities and abuse of medical governance against overseas consultants in Urology Department

Dear ███
Kindly see this email trail. Mr Peter Duffy was a bully and was referred to the management to investigate his behaviour.

From: ███████ (UHMB)
Sent: 16 January 2015 14:57
To: ▓A▓ ███████ (UHMB)
Subject: RE: Harasment,discrimination,unequal opportunities and abuse of medical governance against overseas consultants in Urology Department

Dear Mr ▓A▓

Thank you for forwarding these to me. Can I ask that we catch up after the meeting with ███████ to agree how we proceed.

Regards
███

hello my name is...

███████
███████ ███████ ███████
Surgery & Critical Care
University Hospitals of Morecambe Bay Foundation Trust
Westmorland General Hospital
Burton Road
Kendal
LA9 7RG
☎ ███████
✉ ██████@mbht.nhs.uk

From: ▓A▓ ███████ (UHMB)
Sent: 16 January 2015 11:28
To: ███████ (UHMB)
Subject: FW: Harasment,discrimination,unequal opportunities and abuse of medical governance against overseas consultants in Urology Department
Importance: High

From: ██ ████████ (UHMB) <█████.█ █@mbht.nhs.uk>
Sent: 13 November 2019 17:42
To: ████████
Subject: FW: Confidential

Importance: High
Sensitivity: Confidential

Dear ██
I had received this email from██ who was involved in the investigations of bullying and harassment against Asian consultants by Mr Peter Duffy

From: ██ ████████ (UHMB)
Sent: 10 January 2015 12:45
To: ██ ████████ (UHMB)
Subject: FW: Confidential
Importance: High
Sensitivity: Confidential

From: ████████ ██ (UHMB)
Sent: 09 January 2015 12:52
To: ██ ████████ (UHMB)
Subject: Confidential
Importance: High
Sensitivity: Confidential

Dear Mr ██

As discussed today at the meeting with ████ ████████, please find my mobile number below. You did raise concerns regarding dignity at work and I stated that the Trust takes very seriously any allegations raised. It was agreed that given the work being undertaken by████ (mediation) in January 15 we would review the situation again after this first meeting in January before taking any action.

However please do ring or email me if you have any further concerns or wish to discuss prior to the meeting with ████ in January.

Regards

hello my name is...

██ ████████
██ ████████ ████ ██
Surgery & Critical Care

Clearly, not only had both the police allegations and minutes of the covert meeting where I'd been named and labelled as a racist and bully been extensively circulated around the senior management and executives of UHMBT including the HR department (just as I'd feared, but had been unable to prove to the employment tribunal), but Mr Madhra had secured the minutes of the meeting where, as above, I was named, and was clearly intending to use all these covert briefings to put pressure on the UHMBT non-executive directors about me.

Not only had I been left in complete ignorance of this secret but comprehensive campaign of late 2014 and early 2015, but all this documentation, now revealed in consultant A's voluminous GMC complaint, would have been absolutely critical and pivotal evidence to the employment tribunal, demonstrating that exactly the same allegations as had been made to the police had clearly been circulated and repeated around the senior executives and non-executives of UHMBT. Yet this had all been illegally concealed from the judicial process by the NHS until these explosive allegations had emerged some 18 months later.

How many times did we ask for complete disclosure of exactly this kind of thing? I recalled. And what a massive difference it might have made to the tribunal outcome if all the evidence had been declared, as required by the law, and the panel had been truthfully and properly informed about the extent of the briefings and covert retaliatory campaign against me from within the NHS?

...Instead, all of this was completely concealed from the tribunal and the legal process.

UHMBT had, during the tribunal hearing, given the impression that, if there had been any allegations of prejudice or bullying within the department, these had been low key, generic and non-specific, never really gaining any traction. Clearly, the real truth couldn't have been further away from the sanitised and deceptive version given to the tribunal. Not only had senior managers and non-executive directors been involved, and clearly been responsive to such allegations, but it was equally clear that, in other correspondence, covert discussions had also been had with the UHMBT whistleblowing guardian and bullying champion (who, of course, reported back to UHMBT executives and non-executive directors), and even with the investigators due to conduct the forthcoming 2015 external psychology review of the urology department – the review which preceded my hurried removal from Royal Lancaster Infirmary to Furness General Hospital.

And these were just the very few emails that Mr A had decided to include in his evidence to the GMC. Almost certainly the tiny tip of a huge iceberg. How much more evidence had been concealed from the employment tribunal and was still not known about?

With UHMBT having concealed a good number of potentially pivotal emails from any legal scrutiny by myself, my own legal team and the tribunal, it was difficult, I mused, to avoid the conclusion that another fundamental act of contempt of court had taken place some two years earlier. Potentially, Judge Franey's and the Manchester Employment Tribunal panel's time and effort, deliberations and conclusions had been comprehensively and deliberately invalidated and undermined by this withholding of core evidence, and rendered utterly null and void.

THE GMC AIMS to complete its investigations as quickly as possible and to complete all investigations, as far as possible, within 12 months.

Nevertheless, this was to hang over me for another awful 15 months, despite the laughable lack of any credible evidence, and despite the clear recommendations of the Hooper report from 2015.

Such allegations clearly could not go unanswered. The normal course of events would have been to involve my medical defence organisation (the Medical Protection Society or MPS), but the allegations seemed so random, ridiculous and utterly lacking in evidence and credibility that I thought I'd save them the effort and expense and simply reply myself. Looking back, this was probably a mistake, but one that I thought I'd got away with at the time. Needless to say, I refuted all the allegations.

For the purposes of medical learning, even the most comical and clearly retaliatory GMC allegations should be immediately reported to your medical indemnity provider. Had I done so, I might have saved myself several months of stress and anxiety, and yet more allegations to come.

Only in March 2021 was the case finally closed, more than fifteen months after the initial notification.

Clearly, the GMC still has much to learn about revenge-reporting.

And whilst I might have got away without involving the MPS in 2019, the events of 2020 soon demonstrated the overwhelming need for any potential NHS whistleblower to have comprehensive legal cover. Much, much worse was to follow.

5 March 2021

In reply please quote: GE/C1-2451416468

General Medical Council

Private: Addressee Only
Dr Peter Duffy

Sent by email to: mrpmduffy@

3 Hardman Street
Manchester M3 3AW

Email: gmc@gmc-uk.org
Website: www.gmc-uk.org
Telephone: 0161 923 6602
Fax: 0161 923 6201

Dear Dr Duffy

The case examiners have concluded this case with no further action.

I am writing to update you on the outcome of our review.

The case examiners have considered the information provided by ▇ ▇▇▇▇ ▇ and decided to conclude this case with no further action.

We do understand that this type of enquiry is stressful. I am grateful for your help in putting together all of the information the case examiners needed to make their decision.

Case examiners are senior GMC staff, appointed to make decisions on cases at the end of our review of your fitness to practise. All decisions on cases are made by two case examiners, one is medically qualified and the other case examiner is lay. They took into consideration all of the information that we had gathered and the comments that you made.

The reasons given by the case examiners for their decision are enclosed in **Annex A.**

CHAPTER SIX

Board Meeting

DESPITE ALL THESE DRAMAS, 2019 still wasn't quite finished with me yet. I hadn't managed to attend the UHMBT public Council of Governors meeting that followed shortly after publication of *Whistle in the Wind*, but, in any case, NHS Trust governor's public meetings with the board and non-executives are usually anodyne affairs anyway, attended by few, if any, members of the public and with good reason. Normally, I'd prefer to crawl naked over broken glass and rusty barbed wire rather than spend an afternoon in one, but on the other hand, September's meeting had proved unusually lively, being attended by some 30 members of the public and with several copies of *Whistle in the Wind* being produced. It seemed worth purchasing a day-return ticket via *Fly-Be Maybe* and getting myself over for the next meeting of 10th December 2019, armed with pre-submitted questions for the executives, non-executive directors and governors.

I'd fully expected to either be refused entry to the meeting, or to have my question disallowed but, credit where it's due, UHMBT's council of governors allowed me to submit and read aloud my series of questions. Given such an opportunity, I was determined to present my case as powerfully as possible. Clearly pre-warned about my presence and despite me having showered, shaved and put on a clean, fresh shirt, socks etc. that morning, at least one member of the board got up, moved away from me and took their seat on the opposite side of the room when I sat down.

I was accompanied by Amy Fenton, as well as Karen and Nicola, Peter Read's daughters.

Standing up in front of a hostile and high-powered meeting and reading out a deeply contentious series of questions to my powerful ex-employer was always going to be challenging in the extreme and I remain deeply grateful to them for making the effort to come and support me.

Ladies and Gentlemen…

The problems with a small number of consultants in the urology department are now well known and an external review of these issues is due. However, there remain safety-critical issues which the governors need to hold the board to account over, if the board is to regain the full confidence of staff and patients, regardless of any protracted and drawn-out external enquiry.

Firstly, how was it possible that a consultant surgeon, widely if not universally regarded as dangerous and dysfunctional, was allowed to survive and prosper within the department for nearly two decades, despite the Chief Executive telling me in 2003 that, had I behaved the same, I'd have been sacked 18 months earlier?

How was it that when standards deteriorated again some 7 to 8 years ago, I was instructed by Mr ▮ that incidents must not be formally reported but only fed back by word of mouth, in order to avoid compromising and embarrassing the Trust, despite the avoidable death of Mrs Irene Erhart from inadequately treated sepsis in the meantime?

At the beginning of 2015 we had another avoidable death. Mr Peter Read, yet there was still no Serious Incident or Morbidity & Mortality review. How was it possible that, after the coroner then _ordered_ discussion of Mr Read's case in the M&M meeting, two consultants were allowed to refuse these orders, disobey NHS protocol, sabotage the coroner's investigations and get away with a blatant act of contempt of court and cover-up? How was it that the medical hierarchy _AND_ legal office knew of this disobedience and allowed it to go unchallenged? How was it that, without my knowledge or permission, the coroner was led to believe that I was now favouring an RCA meeting over the coroner's original orders, when the opposite was the truth?

And how was it that for 3 years, the Read family were kept entirely in the dark about this cover-up?

Turning to myself, how was it that a committed surgeon and whistle-blower, UHMBT's Doctor of the Year, was subject to a campaign of vilification, intimidation, lies and covert defamatory comments, <u>still</u> going on in your internal email system today, ultimately having to leave my base hospital to escape from the rudeness, bullying and abuse? And in particular, how could the board have allowed me to be covertly labelled as a fraudster, racist and bully by the very people whose malpractice I had exposed?

After I spoke with the CQC, how was it possible that within months I'd been dismissed, with £35,000 illegally stolen from my earnings, further prospective and retrospective pay cuts, demotion, further detriment and threatened disciplinary action?

And yet, still, the bullying, abuse, threats and harassment has continued, pursuing me all the way into an employment tribunal and now into yet another GMC investigation into my fitness to practice, with utterly false and fabricated allegations including fraud, racism, falsifying notes, bullying, cocaine abuse, amphetamine abuse and alcohol abuse whilst being on duty, to name but a few. How was it that in that employment tribunal, evidence was withheld, emails redacted, potential witnesses forced out, a vital witness statement concealed and life changing six-figure costs threatened, even when I was under oath?

How does this treatment and my and my family's ongoing torture fit with the Trust's legal obligations and the board's promises...<u>promises</u>...of no detriment or dismissal to a whistleblower?

And after all the covert briefings, cover-ups and misleading statements, how does this fit with the Trust's duty of candour, particularly to the bereaved families?

What are NHS staff across the country to make of the fact that after bullying and abuse, resignations, near misses, avoidable deaths, serious and avoidable harm, disobedience to the coroner, threats, lies, retaliation, harassment, broken promises, cover-ups, covert briefings and misleading statements, true to form, the only member of staff to suffer financial punishment and detriment, demotion, dismissal and separation from family and friends is, of course, the NHS whistleblower?

After such a litany of failure, risk taking and cover-up how on earth can these events possibly sit alongside the NHS constitution, freedom to speak up, equality and diversity, and making the NHS a great place to work and to be cared for?

And lastly. Integrity, selflessness, objectivity, leadership, accountability, openness, honesty. All Nolan principles for public life. Would the governors agree that the board has failed to adhere to a single one of these principles in its dealings with the urology department and its patients, staff, bereaved families and myself?'

Sitting down, there was a long silence from the 25 to 30 executive board members, non-executives, governors and members of the public around the room. With the previous chair having abruptly resigned after the previous public meeting, it fell to Liz Sedgley, acting chair of UHMBT, to thank me for attending the meeting.

It can't have been easy for her....

To hear you speak such moving words in person is very powerful.... I can only apologise for what you and your family and the patients have gone through. It wasn't right....

It didn't really address UHMBT's broken-and-then-deleted board promise to its staff of *no detriment or dismissal to any whistleblower,* nor did it go any distance at all towards compensating the family and myself for the years of pain, separation, intimidation and financial penalties inflicted upon us, or addressing the years still to come. But there seemed to be some genuine remorse, at least from some quarters within UHMBT.

Leaving before the meeting was over, I got a nod from Aaron Cummins, Chief Executive; and either averted eyes or stony-faced glares from most of the other attendees. Still, I'd hopefully made my point.

Needless to say, nobody made any coherent attempt to address my last five paragraphs.

They still haven't.

CHAPTER SEVEN

Second RCA

AS WELL AS THE DISTRACTION of the opening of another GMC enquiry into my conduct, the last few weeks of 2019 were characterised by, amongst other things, back-and-forth correspondence between myself, UHMBT and Peter Read's family, *Patient A* from *Whistle in the Wind*.

Amidst all the issues that the book had thrown up, one of the main ones was the original inadequate UHMBT RCA (Root Cause Analysis) investigation into Peter Read's death from 2015 and the response to such an avoidable death from sepsis. As we headed out of 2019 and Christmas and into 2020 and a new year, some five years on from these events, a new and improved RCA was at last, also on the cards.

Tragically and, in my opinion, entirely avoidably, Peter Read had died on the second day of 2015. There was, as far as I could tell, initially no response at all to Mr Read's death from within UHMBT's critical care division or executive during the early months of that year, and certainly no attempt from management or the medical hierarchy to find out if things had gone wrong and what might be improved. Looking back, this was at least in part my fault, something that I deeply regret and accept full responsibility for.

There can be no doubt whatsoever that I should have submitted another formal *clinical incident* about Mr Read's death during the late winter and spring months of 2015. However, it was clear to me, and to others in the department that I had already attracted much adverse attention from my previously expressed concerns (Part I, chapter 5). At this point I wasn't even remotely aware of the covert meetings over racism and bullying allegations, nor the involvement of the BMA and BAPIO (the British Association of Physicians of Indian Origin) in these accusations, but with the unmissable daily hostility towards me, the tip-off in around February that I'd been reported to the police for racism and the fact that UHMBT had organised an external psychological review of the *dysfunctional department*, I (wrongly) told myself that it might be better all-round if I kept my head down over this latest disaster and waited for the inevitable inquest. Perhaps either HM coroner or the external clinical psychologists would show sufficient curiosity to force some safety changes and improvements in clinical behaviour, without me having to stick my neck out even further?

Predictably, Peter Read's avoidable death culminated in the formal coroner's inquest of May 2015. The details are contained in chapter 11 of *Whistle in the Wind* and need not be revisited here in any great detail. However, it seemed clear that with dramatically deteriorating blood tests, including significantly worsening kidney function and 'septic markers' from early Saturday 27th December onwards, Mr Read's overdue-for-change ureteric stent (an artificial tube enabling urine to drain from the kidney down to the bladder) had both blocked, causing an obstructed kidney (as evidenced by the dramatic deterioration in his kidney function blood tests) and become infected with systemic sepsis (as demonstrated by the dramatic rise in his septic blood-markers on the 27th). Yet, despite worsening ward observations, he hadn't made it to theatre for an emergency stent change (thereby allowing the kidney to drain again and the antibiotics to take effect) for another three days.[4] Tragically, although Mr Read initially seemed to rally after I'd found out about the deterioration and rushed him to theatre on the 30th, he never regained consciousness and died, still on the ICU in the early days of

---

[4] Sepsis in the presence of an obstructed kidney is a very urgent surgical emergency, as detailed in *Whistle in the Wind* chapter 10, and the Royal College of Surgeons publication. https://www.rcseng.ac.uk/library-and-publications/rcs-publications/docs/emergency-surgery-standards-for-unscheduled-care/

2015. The coroner had gone on to list sepsis as a major contributory factor in his death.

Complicating matters still further, I'd seen Peter Read myself, on the Friday 26th, the day <u>before</u> his blood tests had deteriorated so dramatically.

Peter had already been on the ward for some weeks under the care of the general surgical team with fluctuating and intermittent bowel obstruction which they were trying to manage conservatively (without resorting to more major bowel surgery).

Telephoned that day of the 26th by the surgical ward staff and asked if there was anyone on-call from the urology team who could speak to Mr Read's family about expediting his already overdue-for-change ureteric stent operation whilst he was still in hospital, I'd gone along later that Friday Boxing Day late afternoon, bumping into his family in the corridor between wards 33 and 34. Agreeing with the family that it made perfect sense to reschedule the relatively low-key endoscopic surgery for whilst Peter was still in hospital under the care of the general surgical team and that we should try and bring the operation forward to early the following week, I'd then gone on to the ward to speak to Mr Read myself. All I remember is a man who, despite clearly being unwell from his intermittent bowel obstruction, was courageous enough to manage at least one very funny joke despite his predicament and who was very grateful that I'd offered to turn in on a bank holiday afternoon to speak to him and his family. With Peter Read happy and clear with our revised plan of theatre on either the following Monday afternoon or Tuesday, I'd emailed the surgical waiting list office, asking them to add Peter to the operating lists for one of these two days, documented it in the notes and headed off home.

I'd been briefly questioned on the events of that day by HM coroner, some months later.

Peter Read's routine ward observations that day had been low risk, and his blood results were normal or near normal (if indeed I'd even checked them, bearing in mind that I hadn't been asked to assess his overall clinical condition). Indeed, his results were exactly what might have been expected under the circumstances. He himself seemed reasonably cheerful if frail, again, entirely consistent with his ongoing general surgical condition. There was no need to do anything other than document the family's concerns about Mr Read's weight loss and poor progress from his conservative bowel obstruction management, ensure that the nursing staff were aware of the plan for an expedited endoscopic stent change early the following week and make sure that I'd documented that I'd sent the request for an expedited operation by email.

Ms Hammond, HM coroner, had closed her cross-examination of my evidence at Mr Read's inquest in 2015 by, in front of his family, questioning me about how a departmental consensus might be sought regarding the events surrounding Peter's last days. Specifically, she wanted the urology department to address, as a group, whether there might have been opportunities prior to the 30th December 2014 (the day of Mr Read's hastily arranged emergency surgery at my hands) but after the deterioration of early on the 27th December to get Mr Read to theatre for his emergency stent replacement. The events of Sunday 28th had clearly caught her attention (by this point, as well as the on-call urology surgeon and general surgical team, the on-call microbiology consultant had now also become involved in the case, the latter advising immediate urological surgery to change the stent).

The contradiction between the clear and escalating concerns of the general surgical team and the advice in favour of immediate emergency surgery that day from the consultant microbiologist; and on the other hand, the actual outcome which was, in fact, no attempt at emergency surgery for nearly another two days was clearly something that troubled Ms Hammond.

She'd asked me, point-blank, if I myself would have taken Mr Read to theatre had I been the on-call urological surgeon that day (the 28th), based upon his observations, clinical condition and dramatically worse blood results over the previous 36 hours.

Under oath, there was only one possible answer.

An unhesitating 'yes' which, with Peter Read's family present at the back, had led to a long silence in the coroner's court.

Ms Hammond had responded by asking me for information about the most appropriate forum for a departmental discussion of Mr Read's case, and particularly a urology departmental consensus and statement from UHMBT's urological surgery specialists on whether his emergency surgery might have been scheduled more expediently. The clear, obvious and indeed only honest answer was that his case should be discussed in our urology Morbidity and Mortality meeting.

M&M meetings, as they are known, have been a key component of the Royal College of Surgeons' 'Good Surgical Practice' since 2014. By the summer of 2015, as referred to in *Whistle in the Wind*, they had already been a longstanding and regular feature of the urology department of UHMBT under the leadership of Colin Cutting, the-then departmental lead. Colin, having instituted these, in turn, had appointed one of my ex-colleagues—consultant B to be the 'M&M lead'. For this he received a time and salary allowance to allow him to collect all the data and prepare and introduce each and all of our departmental cases of deaths or complications over the previous month.

Acknowledging the regular and well established presence of such meetings, Ms Hammond asked me during the inquest if Mr Read's case had already been registered for discussion in the four or five meetings that had followed his death.

It hadn't.

At the time, I'd cringed and braced myself for the obvious question *Why not...?* To which I didn't, in all honesty, have a justifiable answer. However, Ms Hammond had simply proceeded to formally order that Peter Read's case be addressed at the next meeting. She gave me a few weeks to write back with a report detailing the departmental consensus. On accepting that the meetings were held monthly and the last meeting had just occurred, she agreed to extending the deadline for compliance with her order until a few days after the next meeting.

As detailed in *Whistle in the Wind*, on the day of the next M&M meeting, my two ex-colleagues who were on call over that fateful weekend and following Monday both refused to co-operate with the coroner's order and with established surgical *Good Practice*.

*We are not discussing that case...*was the order when I reminded them of HM coroner's instructions and produced Mr Read's notes at the next M&M meeting a few weeks later. This didn't leave much room for compromise, particularly when the response was forcibly repeated despite my protests, and the order not to discuss the case came from Mr B, the-then Morbidity and Mortality lead. The refusal was then followed, after the meeting, by what I considered to be a rather tricky email which seemed to try and spread the blame for the act of coronial disobedience around all four of the consultants who had witnessed the exchange, implying that we'd all agreed together to disobey the coroner.

The remaining manoeuverings are described in more detail in chapter 11 of *Whistle in the Wind*, including the relevant email correspondence. Unsurprisingly and entirely predictably, the subsequent Root Cause Analysis (RCA) report, hurriedly put into place by UHMBT after the act of coronial disobedience and completely lacking in any independent and specialist urological surgery input, was roundly and entirely correctly rejected by the coroner. Expressing my own disbelief about what I considered to be a wilful act of coronial disobedience, possible contempt of court, a cover-up over an avoidable death and ongoing risk-taking to the Care Quality Commission in late summer of 2015 (at roughly the same time that HM coroner rejected the RCA report), the UHMBT hierarchy was, by this point, acutely aware of both my own concerns and those of the coroner.

Yet this flawed, biased and rejected RCA report, unequivocally rebuffed and rejected by HM coroner, by myself and by at least one other senior urological surgeon, was nevertheless presented to Peter Read's family that Autumn of 2015 as an explicit statement of fact and allowed to remain on the record for more than another four years. Only in late 2019, and only after the furore created by the book, the local MPs, and both Amy Fenton's and Mr Read's family's persistent questioning, was there finally any attempt to revisit a report that had formally remained as a definitive, accurate and faithful NHS record of events, despite been roundly rejected years earlier by none other than HM coroner herself.

———————

BUT, AT LAST AND NEARLY FIVE YEARS after Mr Read's avoidable death and the coroner's subsequent order came signs of change. Correspondence between Mr Read's family, UHMBT and myself went back and forth and in late 2019, there seemed at last to be signs of willingness to properly address what had happened. Peter Read's entire family had witnessed HM coroner's order in the Lancaster Coroner's Court of 2015 about departmental discussion and the need for an M&M meeting and consensus, and were persistent in pointing out that, more than four years on, this order still hadn't been obeyed.

After much correspondence, UHMBT reluctantly agreed to start the process again *from scratch*. Although another RCA was mooted, rather than the M&M discussion ordered by the coroner, we were all assured that an external urological surgeon would preside over the process and, with the process starting *from scratch*, there would at long last be a proper impartial evaluation of the facts. New witness reports would clearly need to be commissioned from the relevant participants, and the original ones, subject to such an unfair and prejudiced process of collection (as described in *Whistle in the Wind*, page 105) would clearly have to be discarded. As we headed into Christmas, although there was still no M&M discussion and therefore no prospect of the letter of the coroner's legal orders being fulfilled, we did at least seem to have some progress.

In late 2019 I was still waiting to provide my new *start from scratch* witness statement to the fresh RCA meeting. Questioning when my new statement would be required, to my utter disbelief and astonishment, I was informed that this wouldn't be necessary. Information Governance at UHMBT had decided that, despite the assurances to both Mr Read's family and myself that the process would be *started from scratch*, someone had quietly but clearly gone back on the original assurances and decided that the new RCA report should be, once again, based on the original statements, despite the biased and unfair way in which they'd been collected, and the fact that the Trust knew all along that they'd been collected in a biased and unfair way.

Repeatedly arguing for new statements, both I and Peter Read's family were overruled and told that the new report would be based upon the clinical notes and the old, original witness statements, collected in 2015.

Once again, to my despair, we'd gone back to the original, tainted and unfairly collected statements. Peter Read's family and I were incredulous that, once again, skewed evidence would be put to Professor Ian Pearce, the external expert opinion. It also seemed likely that Professor Pearce wouldn't be made aware that my ex-colleagues A and B had seemingly collaborated and exchanged personal statements in 2015, suggested modifications to each other and been able to modify or add to their statements again, after being shown my own evidence to the coroner.

Of course, I'd been offered no opportunities to take such liberties with my own evidence.

With both statements making allegations and containing implications (particularly relating to the Friday 26th December) which I'd never been allowed to respond to, the stage seemed to me to be set for yet another potential cover-up and attempt to shift responsibility.

RECEIVING THE PRELIMINARY REVISED RCA DRAFT in late December 2019, whilst it was clear that the report was considerably more rigorous and thorough than the original report of 2015, once more and entirely predictably, a number of misinterpretations had crept into the text. A major error, directly as a consequence of using the original, misleading statements was that, once again, it appeared to be unequivocally accepted that Peter Read had been formally referred across to me as an emergency by the general surgical team on the Friday 26th, thus clearly implying that I should have formally surgically assessed Peter, potentially taken over his care and possibly even arranged for emergency surgery that Friday evening. The truth, of course, was that, as above, I'd simply attended the ward as a courtesy, following a low-key, non-urgent request, passed on from one of the ward staff for someone from the urology team, if available, to come and speak to the family about expediting Mr Read's planned regular stent change. The first of the dramatic changes in Peter Read's blood markers that was to trigger appropriate alarm in the general surgical team and a subsequent attempt to involve the on-call urology consultant was still some twelve hours away and into the future....

All of this could have been avoided if UHMBT had stuck to their original assurances that those involved would be asked to provide new statements, on this occasion drawn up in accordance with fair and judicial standards of practice and protocol.

———————

THE NEW RCA REPORT was due to be discussed in a face-to-face meeting at UHMBT headquarters in Kendal in the second week of January 2020.

Taking a day's annual leave to fly over and back again is extremely stressful, exhausting and expensive, as I'd already learned several times over from previous meetings, but I had an overwhelmingly powerful sense that if I wasn't there, then there'd be a determined attempt to gloss over elements of the story, possibly spin out new versions and dramatically play up any aspects that reflected badly on myself. Wearily, I committed myself to the expense of another day's annual leave and the cost of travel to and from Kendal (UHMBT's headquarters), via Manchester and Ballasalla Airport.

It was a very good decision indeed. The meeting, held mid-afternoon, was indeed extremely stressful, not least having to go back and sit around the table with two ex-colleagues who, I felt, had played such a major role in my unfair and illegal dismissal from UHMBT. Despite taking a significant dose of my prescribed beta-blockers beforehand, I still couldn't keep my ventricular ectopics (irregular heartbeats) under control and, by the end of the meeting, had a headache bad enough to worry me that I might have had a stroke.

Opening the meeting, and possibly aware of my, and Peter Read's family's frustrations over the use of the original statements in the new RCA, Professor Pearce made the case for basing the new report on the old statements rather than collecting new ones, pointing out, perfectly reasonably, that it would be remarkable if anyone could recall anything different from five years earlier, over and above their original statements.

Very presciently indeed, he also noted that it would be extremely irregular for a witness to give a statement for the purposes of the coroner, and then, five years down the line, significantly change, alter or backtrack on that statement, thereby potentially perjuring themselves.

Nevertheless, I had a sick feeling that this was exactly what might be about to happen.

Supplied with only the original, biased statements Professor Pearce, perfectly understandably, had clearly formed the impression that I had been formally called out to the ward on the Boxing Day Friday to review Peter Read in response to an emergency summons from the general surgical team.

After five years of spin and cover-up and of being subject to repeated attempts to force-feed to me this fundamental misrepresentation of events, by this point I was extremely angry and unable to stop this showing. My responses were largely read out from a statement that I'd drafted the previous evening.

> *Putting all this together* (the latest RCA implication that I had formally been called to see Peter Read on the 26th December after an emergency referral from the general surgeons), *it would seem to be a prima facie example of gross neglect and negligence, even possibly involuntary manslaughter.*
>
> *Undoubtedly, the first and greatest error leading to the avoidable death of Peter Read was mine.*
>
> *…Or it would be, if the clinical scenario that I have just painted for you were anything other than a blatant frame-up….*

*So, after 4½ years, let's be <u>absolutely clear</u> here. Once, and for all and for the record. Peter Read was <u>**never**</u> referred across to me by the general surgeons on Friday, 26th December 2014...and everything that subsequently flows from that central deceit is false.*

*The general surgeons did a ward round that morning...(the 26th). They were clearly thinking about discharging Mr Read (sending him home). I can categorically state that at no point that day was there <u>**any**</u> urgent referral or call for advice or anything from the general surgical team...the call did <u>**not**</u> come from the general surgical team but from the family, via the ward staff. Mr Read's family were visiting and had asked if there was anyone in the hospital that could speak to them about Mr Read and whether his elective (non-urgent) urological stent change date could be brought forward.*

MY VIGOROUS AND ABSOLUTE REJECTION of the version of events inferred in the accounts given by my two previous colleagues of the 26th, now, once again, incorporated into this latest RCA draft, didn't go down at all well, with clear dismay around much of the table and one senior executive muttering *this is exactly where I didn't want to find us....*

As it turned out, had I not taken the trouble to travel over that day and put the true version of events, then it seems clear that the final report would have concluded that Peter Read had been formally referred to me by the general surgical team on the 26th as an emergency and as a case of possible urinary tract sepsis. Therefore, each and every one of the subsequent catastrophic and ultimately lethal events was, seemingly, a domino effect triggered by my initial failure to diagnose and act upon Peter Read's sepsis (which in actual fact didn't declare itself until the following day).

Thankfully, having made the decision to attend and reading from my prepared notes I was comprehensively able to reject this.

No one tried any further to argue the case for Peter's sepsis and stent obstruction having presented on the 26th.

Moving on to the events of the following weekend and Monday, once again I was aghast at the attempts to rewrite what had gone on and attempts to backdate a new version of events into the record.

Mr A had taken over the on-call responsibility for urological surgery from myself on the morning of the 27th December. He'd repeatedly and vigorously claimed in his original statement for the coroner in 2015 that Peter Read hadn't needed to go to theatre for an emergency replacement of his overdue-for-change stent over that fateful weekend, despite being phoned for advice by the general surgical team on the 27th, and despite, 24 hours later, Peter being formally referred across to Mr A as an emergency on the 28th. This was, of course, a couple of days after I'd seen Mr Read myself, and by this point the blood results early on the 27th were clearly indicating a huge jump in his septic markers, as well as a very significant deterioration in his kidney function. With Peter's overall condition unmistakably deteriorating significantly over the weekend, the on-call urological surgeon had seemingly dismissed the concerns of both the general surgeons and microbiologist that day of the 28th, despite the emergency referral and had clearly made the point that Mr Read did not need emergency surgery and could safely wait until a regular operating list the following week.

The screenshots below are taken from the weekend on-call urological surgeon's original statement of June 2015, which was in turn used to inform both the original RCA report to HM coroner and this latest RCA report, and which was also incorporated into the legal bundle as evidence to the employment tribunal of Mr A's position on the events of the 28th.

I spoke to the anaesthetic ICU registrar as well as Dr   consultant Anaesthetist ICU for their opinion. They found the patient not suitable for the ICU Based on the clinical findings and the investigations. They adviced that patient should continue the same treatment in the ward. They said that patient will need stent change at **some point**. They did not feel that immediate change was needed and hence the plan to get the stent change under care of Mr Duffy early next week stayed the same.

On the basis of current findings stent change was not deemed urgently necessary and this is the routine course of action for all urology patients. At this stage patient was stable , showing signs of improvement and no obvious sepsis. In the hind sight it is easy to make decisions but as clinicians we have to decide on the day itself. I had taken the advice from two other specialists and we all agreed to the plan of action on that day.

I believe that the patient received good clinical care and attention from me on 28/12/14 when I was called to see the patient. There were no clinical indication to press on the emergency change of the stent on that day. I had discussed the situation with the ICU registrar as well as the ICU consultant.

I feel satisfied with my handling of this patient on 28/12/14 and a joint decision was taken. The patient was improving and there was no indication for an emergency stent change on that day.

Silently recalling Professor Pearce's comments about changes in evidence to the coroner and the potential for perjuring oneself, I was dumbfounded to hear Mr A carry out what appeared to be a screeching, tyre-smoking U-turn in his evidence. Faced with the meeting, and particularly Professor Pearce stating their collective opinion that Peter Read should have gone to theatre for immediate and mandatory emergency surgery on the Sunday (as advised by the consultant microbiologist at the time), suddenly and out of the blue, Mr A protested and maintained, in what appeared to be a complete contradiction of his original statements provided both for the coroner and forwarded to Manchester Employment Tribunal, that he had indeed believed at the time that Peter required emergency surgery that day. Indeed, he had been clear on the need to take Peter to theatre on the 28th for an emergency change of his ureteric stent all along. However, it was his consideration that Mr Read's deterioration by that time meant that he was now too sick to risk an anaesthetic and emergency surgery without intensive care (ICU) backup.

Mr A went on to claim that he'd been informed that Peter Read wasn't unwell enough at this point for admission to the ICU. Furthermore, he'd been informed that ICU was full and was two patients over capacity. Therefore, with a sick patient requiring emergency surgery but no ICU bed available, it was his judgement that, although emergency surgery was, after all, indicated that afternoon, it was too hazardous to attempt any interventions and the emergency surgery would basically have to wait for some other time and some other consultant surgeon the following week.

Professor Pearce fundamentally disagreed with this, pointing out that it was indeed a risk to push for surgery, but a much greater risk to simply delay and put off emergency intervention, with the clear potential for the patient to deteriorate further. He also pointed out that there was nothing in the notes about there being no available ICU bed. Nevertheless, Mr A was adamant that he had pressed his case for ICU admission as a prelude to his plans for emergency surgery that day, even going so far, he claimed, as walking over to the ICU department to negotiate with them and see if there was any possibility of a bed being generated to accommodate Peter Read if required. With no possibility of a patient being exchanged or any space being cleared on ICU for Mr Read if needed post-operatively, my ex-colleague's new position was that emergency surgery was indicated, but could not proceed over the weekend as Peter was not fit enough, and that he would therefore simply have to wait for the emergency procedure.

In a later written response to the new RCA report, which subsequently and dutifully incorporated this radically new and contradictory evidence, I wrote:

> In respect to the afternoon management (of Peter Read on the 28th) that involved Mr A being called into the hospital, the original

statement by him (contained on page 629 of the legal bundle) suggests that changing Mr Read's stent was not deemed to be urgently necessary and that the plan was for the change of stent to be carried out under my care later the following week. However, it would now appear from Professor Pearce's RCA that a separate pre-RCA meeting communication from Mr A...claimed that in fact Mr A had wanted to take Peter Read to theatre but there was no available bed on intensive care....

This is the first time, after five years, that this allegation has been made and is clearly a contradiction of Mr A's original evidence. It should not be difficult to determine whether there was indeed space in intensive care for Peter Read and whether any attempt was made to get Peter Read to theatre that afternoon. Furthermore, it would be worth looking to see if any of the patients on intensive care that afternoon were actually stable enough to be transferred to the ward to make space for Mr Read.

I went on to detail my own experience of such situations (thankfully rare), when emergency surgery is needed but the patient may require intensive care support post-operatively, and where ICU is full, with no patients in a position to be transferred or *swapped* out for the unfortunate individual requiring immediate surgery.

...I have never, in some four decades of front-line clinical medicine and surgery, come across a situation where a patient requiring emergency surgery has been cancelled because of a lack of an intensive care bed. The principle under these circumstances is that the surgery <u>always</u> goes ahead as quickly as is reasonably possible and if there is no intensive care bed available post operatively then the patient is either held in the recovery bay (where similar facilities to ICU can be used), *transferred to a neighbouring ICU or alternatively a more stable patient would be transferred either to the ward or another facility to make space for the post-operative patient. Of course, if conventional practice had been ignored in this case, then there would have been a huge amount of annotation spread throughout the notes about such an unusual clinical decision....*

There is none.

Overall, my impression here is of the truth not being told. This is serious enough, but for liberties to be taken with the actuality in a very serious case like this, involving an avoidable death and potential serious negligence, attempts to frustrate the coroner's enquiries and indeed potentially mislead the coroner, together with some of the fallout for members of the team after this event, particularly my constructive dismissal and the family being kept in the dark about the true events, I think that any attempt to further pervert and distort the true sequence of events should be taken very seriously indeed.[5]

Astonishingly, there was an attempt to retrospectively rewrite the events of Monday 29th too.

Following on from early afternoon Sunday the 28th December, and despite the clear, ongoing urological emergency situation, Peter Read wasn't seen again by a member of the urology team for another 15 to 20 hours. However, the following morning, another consultant ex-colleague (Mr B, who had, in turn, taken over the on-call responsibility from Mr A), was informed of Peter Read's predicament and deterioration over the weekend. With the ward nurses and urology team appropriately arranging for another ICU review, on this occasion it was agreed that Mr Read had deteriorated still further to the point where he <u>did</u> now need ICU admission and supportive care.

Mr B himself documented that morning that he would organise a CT scan and would arrange to take Mr Read to theatre himself as an emergency as soon as he'd been readied for surgery on the ICU.

However, no CT was ever booked; nor was there any evidence that radiology was ever spoken to. No one appeared to have checked

---

[5] Further clinical evidence, provided later by the Trust under a Freedom of Information request has revealed that on Sunday the 28th December 2014 there was a patient on ICU who was *ward ready*, plus another patient who was also *ward-ready* being held in the operating theatre recovery bay. Both of these ICU patients were waiting for ward beds to become available and could have been very straightforwardly exchanged for Mr Read on that Sunday afternoon, enabling immediate emergency surgery to go ahead with full ICU backup if needed post-operatively.

on Mr Read's condition later that day, nor made any attempt to discuss Peter's predicament with theatres, the ICU staff or the emergency on-call anaesthetist. Importantly, there was also no evidence either of any handover to the next on-call urology consultant who had taken over the on-call duties from Mr B at 6pm that Monday.

Both the ICU notes and the Read family's group recollection were clear that, despite that morning's documented assurances about taking charge of Mr Read's needs for emergency imaging and surgery, the urological surgery plan late on that fateful Monday afternoon and evening was still that of an elective (non-emergency) change of the stent without any scans or imaging on the following day of the 30th.

There was no explanation offered to the RCA meeting as to why the CT scan and emergency theatre intervention had not been booked or carried out on that Monday, as had been documented and planned.

Having remained silent for virtually the entire RCA meeting, on-call consultant urological surgeon B for that Monday suddenly broke into the presentation, stating that in fact, Monday the 29th December was a bank holiday.

To the open mouthed disbelief of all present, the consultant went on to claim that, due to the 29th being a bank holiday Monday, he had just been temporarily covering the on-call commitment for Mr Cutting. Handing over Peter Read's case during or at the end of the shift therefore wasn't his responsibility. Mr B implied that he was therefore not responsible for the lack of action later on that Monday and had only properly taken over the regular daily emergency on call work on the Tuesday, this being the next full working day after the weekend and bank holiday Monday of the 29th.

Glimpsing Ian Pearce shaking his head out of the corner of my eye, this completely new version of events was immediately dismissed as entirely false by everyone present; not least Colin himself.

The 29th was a normal working day. The 25th and 26th had been bank holidays and on the Monday, the regular rota had resumed. The consultant urological surgeon in question had been on call and responsible for organising Mr Read's care and progression to emergency imaging and surgery throughout.

Comprehensively refuting any on call responsibility for the events of the 29th, Colin pointed that we'd no idea who was on call that evening. However, there was clearly no evidence whatsoever of any attempt to organise imaging, emergency theatre intervention, handover or attempt to pass on the gravity of the situation by Mr B, who clearly **was** the on-call surgeon for the day, despite his protests to the contrary.

With no handover, the evening on-call surgeon on that Monday, whoever that might have been, had clearly remained in ignorance of Mr Read's terrible predicament.

At that point, aside from my utter disbelief at the attempt to re-portray the 29th as a bank holiday and blame someone else for the lack of handover, I took no notice whatsoever of this new bit of information. It might have been me on-call; or perhaps one of half a dozen other people who had taken over that evening. However, it was clear that, despite the protestations, there had been no handover to anyone during, or at the end of the day on-call, and it had been left to me to find out about Mr Read's desperate predicament from one of the nurses when I arrived on the surgical ward the next day.

However, these discussions about the lack of handover that evening of the 29th came back to bite me very hard indeed, with a nearly lethal outcome, some six months later.

THE REMAINDER OF THE MEETING passed in a haze of tension, disbelief and an extreme headache.

As someone brought up to simply tell the truth and stick to it, I couldn't believe that I'd just witnessed two attempts to insert entirely new and unsubstantiated versions of events into the report; both designed, in my opinion, to shift responsibility on to others. And this wasn't just any old report. This would be going to the bereaved family and, almost certainly, to HM coroner.

Clearly, in my opinion, the consultant on-call for the Saturday and Sunday was now attempting to place the responsibility squarely on the ICU department. Claiming that Mr Read had been too unwell for surgery without the backup of an ICU bed therefore meant, in this new version of events, that Mr Read's emergency surgery therefore had to be deferred over the weekend and into the following week despite the clear potential; indeed, very high likelihood of further deterioration. The second on-call consultant for that period (Monday 29th) had equally clearly tried and failed to introduce a new version of events where, in fact, responsibility for Mr Read's ongoing care that Monday afternoon and evening rested elsewhere on account of the Monday being a bank holiday, which, of course, it wasn't.

Thank God I'd taken the trouble to travel over and was there to help challenge these attempts to rewrite and backdate events and shift blame onto others. At least, having exposed such tactics and having so vigorously insisted that reports and versions of events should stick to the truth, surely no one would now make any further, more devious attempts to retrospectively rewrite what had gone on and introduce yet more dubious evidence into the process?

CHAPTER EIGHT

The Independent Urology Investigation Niche's First Meeting

AFTER THE CONFUSION AND EXTREME frustrations of the 'new' RCA that had, nevertheless gone back to the old and misleading statements, together with the attempts to introduce new versions of what had gone on over that Christmas 2014 bank holiday weekend and subsequent Monday, the next mountain to climb was the inaugural meeting with Niche Health and Social Care Consulting, the private investigatory organisation selected to carry out NHS England's investigation into the urology issues and the circumstances around my whistleblowing and dismissal.

With our first meeting scheduled for the 14th February 2020, I'd hoped to travel out the evening of the 13th via the Isle of Man Steampacket ferry (Isle of Man Steam-racket to some Manx residents), spend a night with Fiona and the boys and drive down to meet Niche the following morning. In the event, I had to cancel this journey after a call from the Emergency Department at Noble's that afternoon about that ultimate male horror-story...a fractured testicle.

Thankfully, not least for the patient, it all ended happily and, rebooking via an early morning *Fly-Be-Maybe* flight, I managed to get to central Manchester by about 8.30am, completing my journey to Niche's Headquarters with a bracing walk along the towpath of the Bridgewater Way canal. Garnished with sickly green algae and the odd bloated rat-corpse, I wasn't feeling my best by the time I reached the Old Trafford area (probably like the previous evening's patient), but Kate and Mary-Ann, both Niche investigators, were quick to greet me and put me at my ease.

With comfy chairs, coffee, biscuits and sympathy, I quickly recovered my appetite and we spent the morning talking through the issues that had led me to publish *Whistle in the Wind*.

We covered a great deal in that morning's discussions and I was deeply impressed with Kate and Mary-Ann's inside knowledge of the workings of the NHS, the CQC, NHS England and employment tribunals. Both seemed to be extremely sharp, worldly-wise and highly experienced investigators and both had read and were fully conversant with the details of *Whistle in the Wind*, even before Niche had been appointed to head up the NHS England investigation. Additionally, both were, it appeared (at least at the time) deeply sympathetic over what had happened to my vocation, career and, of course, my family and home life.

At last, it seemed, we might get a thorough-going, impartial and fearless investigation that would follow the truth and evidence, rather than automatically siding with the big-bucks and big-battalions.

Exiting Trafford House and sitting at the tram stop enjoying a little late winter sunshine, it seemed that the extra cost of the Flybe flight to make that meeting had been an excellent investment. At last, I had a truly impartial and knowledgeable private investigative organisation involved who would adhere strictly to their Terms of Reference and who would ruthlessly and fearlessly follow the truth and evidence wherever it led them.

CHAPTER NINE

Anonymous Tip-off

MONDAY 24th FEBRUARY 2020 started much like any normal day at Noble's Hospital. Having completed a ward round of our in-patients on wards one and two and with a few minutes to spare before endoscopy, I settled down with Julie in the office to go through the new paperwork. Anonymous amongst the slew of letters and results was an entirely unremarkable looking brown envelope. Postmarked *Manchester* and dated the previous Saturday, the envelope was handwritten in a powerful looking scrawl, but with a rather odd combination of upper and lowercase letters. I opened it without any great thoughts or expectations.

Dear Mr Peter Duffy

Hope you are well.

 I am a nurse. I know you very well. You are a very brave person and have stood up for your patients.

 But have suffered a lot.

 Just to inform you that ▆▆▆▆ *and* ▆▆▆ *have employed 2 staff from band 4 to band 7 and asked them to hide all your files and the concerns that you have raised about the managers and directors. They are also doing this for* ▆▆ ▆▆ ▆▆▆ *is another person involved. They are doing this for CQC so that they don't have access to all these documents and your concerns.*

 ▆▆▆▆ *says –*

 'He had damages us and I will make sure to bring him to court and will not sit until he is jailed'

Wish you well.

Regards

Sorry can't give my name as I am may lose my job.

After a shocked and sickening moment of taking in the full import of this, my private office, ideally with a locked door seemed the place to be. Reading it through again, I was chilled to the core. ██████ *says…. 'I will make sure to bring him to court and will not sit until he is jailed'.*

I knew that I'd generated an awful lot of hatred within certain parts of UHMBT and, in some ways, after the goings-on in the employment tribunal, this anonymous tip-off that evidence was potentially being tampered with didn't particularly surprise me. But being detested enough that at least one powerful individual wouldn't rest until I was incarcerated?

That was genuinely frightening…. And, of course, was likely to involve considerably more than just hiding files and evidence.

Casting my mind back to late 2016, I was reminded of UHMBT's attempts to institute retaliatory legal proceedings against me, claiming that I had invoiced for work when I wasn't in the hospital and the allegations, under oath, that I'd *invoiced for up to £112,340 that I was potentially not entitled to….* Recalling my shock at these particular tactics and the damage already done to me and the family, such a threat about a prison sentence didn't sound out-of-character or particularly exaggerated.

I've erased the names, but the anonymous writer clearly knew their way around UHMBT. A number of senior staff were named, including at least two who are not at all known outside the Trust. Clearly, this wasn't some crank, but was someone who was very familiar with NHS staff banding and the senior UHMB Trust hierarchy.

Getting immediately on the phone to both Niche Consulting and NHS England, I was categorically assured that the tip-off would be treated with the utmost urgency and importance. I fully expected to be informed that there would be an immediate snap inspection of the

Trust, that Niche and NHS England had notified the CQC, police and National Cyber Crime Unit of potential meddling with evidence in an important enquiry into, amongst other things, an avoidable death, and that the named individuals had been immediately excluded from any further contact with potential evidence. Also, expecting to be kept fully informed about ongoing developments, particularly with the gravity of such a threat, I was deeply disappointed.

Chasing things up after a few days, I was blandly informed that the matter was 'in hand' and I'd nothing to be fearful of. The issue was being looked into by a Trust non-executive director, UHMBT had assured NHS England and Niche that all was perfectly well and there was *nothing to see here*. Niche and NHS England had accepted these assurances and there was no more to add.

After a few more days of silence, I got back on the phone. Further enquiries simply resulted in what felt like more evasions and bland platitudes. No one seemed prepared to categorically tell me that the whole letter was a fabrication and a pack of lies, leading, of course, to the suspicion that there was substantial element of truth to the tipoff. However, it was clear that I'd get no further with my concerns that evidence was being tampered with internally and that, at least as far as UHMBT, Niche and NHS England were concerned, the matter was firmly and unequivocally closed.

However, I remain profoundly and forever grateful to the individual who took the personal risk of tipping me off. As events later that year showed, the tip-off was anything but irrelevant. Far from having nothing to worry about, there was in fact, reason to be very fearful indeed.

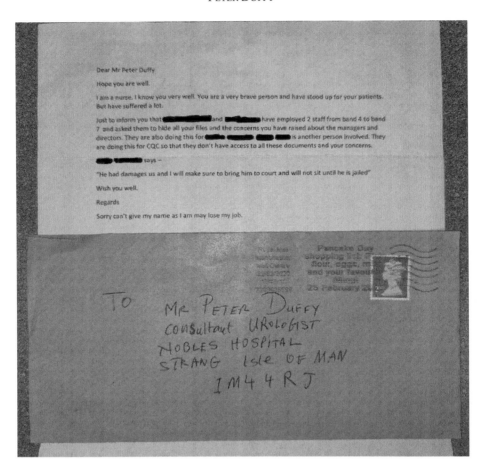

Dear Mr Peter Duffy,

Hope you are well.

I am a nurse. I know you very well. You are a very brave person and have stood up for your patients. But have suffered a lot.

Just to inform you that ██████████ and ████████ have employed 2 staff from band 4 to band 7 and asked them to hide all your files and the concerns you have raised about the managers and directors. They are also doing this for ████ ████ ████ ████ is another person involved. They are doing this for CQC so that they don't have access to all these documents and your concerns.

████ ████ says –

"He had damages us and I will make sure to bring him to court and will not sit until he is jailed"

Wish you well.

Regards

Sorry can't give my name as I am may lose my job.

TO   MR PETER DUFFY
CONSultant UROLOGIST
NOBLES HOSPITAL
STRANG Isle OF MAN
    IM4 4 R J

CHAPTER TEN

Morbidity and Mortality Meeting

IMMEDIATELY AFTER THE RCA PRESENTATION by Professor Pearce in January 2020 (chapter 7) there followed a meeting between UHMBT and Peter Read's family. Not unreasonably, I was excluded from this, but, amongst other things, the report's findings were discussed, with the family confirming, amongst other things, that they and emphatically not the general surgical team had been responsible for me being contacted by the ward staff on that fateful Friday afternoon of the 26th. The family confirmed that I had indeed gone along and discussed expediting Peter Read's elective stent change with them and that there had been no emergency referral to me, or involvement of the general surgical team in my attendance.

Seemingly accepting this version of events, the family were informed by UHMBT that, after this new RCA meeting, HM coroner's instructions of 2015 had now been fulfilled. The case had now been discussed in the urology departmental Morbidity and Mortality meeting and a departmental conclusion reached. That conclusion being that there had indeed been failings across the board in Mr Read's care. From UHMBT's point of view, apologies would now be made, they had discharged their obligations to the coroner and the case was now closed, from the Trust's point of view anyway.

The Read family, quite rightly, were having none of this. Karen and Nicola Read, by this point well aware that a proper M&M meeting comprises a good deal more than an external report and secretive discussions and disagreements behind closed doors, pointed out that this latest meeting by no means got the Trust off the hook. HM coroner had explicitly ordered that a departmental consensus be found, utilising a departmental M&M meeting to do so and by no stretch of the imagination did the previous hour-or-so's presentation, together with shocking and contradictory new facts about the Sunday and Monday from my two ex-colleagues constitute a *departmental consensus*.

Reluctantly, UHMBT conceded that; yes, more than five years on, Peter Read's case should, at last, be discussed, as per the coroner's court order, in an M&M meeting with active participation, learning and input from the rest of the department.

As always happens with the NHS, discussions dragged on to the point that we were deep into the first wave of COVID-19 by the scheduled date for the meeting. With the restrictions, the meeting would have to be held remotely via Microsoft Teams and initially at least, it seemed that neither Professor Alison Birtle (Mr Read's clinical oncologist) or myself were going to be invited to attend. After protests, we were offered an opportunity to dial in.

Very clearly, this was going to be no ordinary M&M meeting, with the Chief Executive, Medical Director, divisional head and divisional lead clinician amongst others all in attendance. Not remotely the sort of atmosphere that was conducive to free, candid and open debate and an arrival at a departmental consensus, as ordered by HM coroner, but I thought I'd let that go past.

However, I wasn't so keen on letting something else go past. Knowing the NHS as well as I do, I fully expected a long, drawn out presentational monologue, followed by a tactically short period for departmental discussion to ensure that as little time as possible was offered for candid and potentially awkward departmental views. It is a well tried and tested NHS tactic, akin to talking out a debate or *filibustering*, thus allowing no opportunity for views that might be uncomfortable or embarrassing.

Sure enough, I sent the following email on the morning of June 4th, the scheduled date of the five-year-late M&M meeting.

From: Duffy, Peter
Sent: 04 June 2020 10:09
To: Shahedal Bari
Cc: Aaron Cummins;

Subject: RE: M & M

Thanks Shahedal

 Yes, I'm well aware of how M&M's work.... The time for discussion seems extraordinarily short. The whole point of an M&M discussion is to allow full and frank discussion ranging over the issues and specialty learning. I usually encourage participants to...take no more than a minute or two to present the salient points, followed by comprehensive discussion for as long as it takes to determine what happened and draw the appropriate learning points. In this case we're going to have an hour-long monologue about a report that we've all read anyway, followed by 15 minutes questions / comments. Perhaps 45 seconds of questions / comments per departmental attendee. Don't you think that this will give the strong impression to the family, Niche and possibly the GMC too that the Trust doesn't want a full, free-ranging and comprehensive discussion to include some of the contradictions and different versions of events contained within Ian's report?

 People have waited for 5 years to discuss and comment on this case which carries all sorts of implications, especially considering my ongoing GMC FTP (fitness to practice) inquiry. The statements within the report appear to validate the original allegations of negligence against myself from 2015 despite the lack of evidence and it'll be a travesty if we don't get the time to fully explore these allegations and insinuations and try and get to the truth of events.

 And, after all, how can we learn and improve if we can't even establish the truth of exactly what happened? I'd suggest that you allocate a lot more time for discussion if this is indeed to be signed off and accepted as a legitimate M&M discussion.

Peter

Entirely unsurprisingly, I was overruled. With the presentation overrunning, as predicted, there was virtually no time for comments and questions from the rest of the department. One new fact that emerged was that it was indeed me who had taken over the urology on-call duties on the Monday evening of the 29th December. However, with no hand over, I'd been left in complete ignorance of Mr Read's plight on ICU until my visit to the surgical ward next morning.

Even as a non-employee and viewed over Microsoft Teams, the meeting came across as tense and intimidating and the only really pertinent observation and question came from Colin Cutting, asking if the consultants involved in Peter Read's care had any observations to make; any learning points and would like to reflect on their role. Quick to jump in and offer my own reflections and regrets to the family, I was firmly overruled and the question was judged to be *inappropriate*.

I sent the following email immediately after the meeting.

From: Duffy, Peter
Sent: 04 June 2020 18:14
To: Shahedal Bari Cc: Aaron Cummins
Subject: RE: M & M

Thanks Shahedal and Aaron
  Disappointing that the department as a whole never got any chance to have their say or to discuss things amongst themselves. That was, of course, the whole thrust of Ms Hammond's (the coroner's) order back in 2015, that a departmental consensus be reached about whether Peter's stent should have been changed before the Tuesday.
  We heard Ian's point of view, which was measured and well-informed, but I felt that we ran out of time far too early, as I feared and predicted, and no one else from the department got to comment.
  Disappointing too that there was no chance for myself, Mr A or Mr B to speak about our own reflective practice or whether we felt that we owed the Read family an apology. I would have liked the chance to do that. Anyway, the two important things came out of this, in my opinion.
  First is Mr A's clear and, I think, repeated statement that he did believe that Peter Read needed emergency surgery on the Sunday and was blocked by no ICU bed, yet at the same time his insistence that there was no evidence that Mr Read had urosepsis. So why did

he need to go to theatre for emergency surgery then? Of course, this also completely contradicts his original statements to the coroner from 2015....

The second thing was Ian's concession that by going over and above my duties and professional obligations, going into the hospital to speak to the family personally about Peter's elective stent change on Boxing Day, and 'going the extra mile'...I actually left myself vulnerable to counter-allegations of neglect and negligence.

What a tragedy that these counter-allegations of negligence from Mr B and Mr A (...completely refuted by the family), all arose out of nothing more than an act of kindness.

Thanks
Peter

UNFORTUNATELY, THAT WAS THE END of the five year battle by the family and myself to get HM coroner's orders obeyed.

There never has been a proper, reflective, constructive and well-chaired Morbidity and Mortality styled discussion, careful departmental learning and debate amongst the UHMBT urological surgeons over Peter Read's death, as ordered by Ms Hammond, Her Majesty's coroner nearly six years ago.

And now, with the family and myself having given up; there never will be.

CHAPTER ELEVEN

Pandemic

LIKE MOST PEOPLE, I began to clock that something was amiss in China sometime in early January 2020. The odd report in the Guardian or Telegraph hinted at something that sounded a good deal worse than seasonal flu, but it was thousands of miles away and would almost certainly fade away, just like the bird-flu media frenzy had done a few years earlier. I was aware, as most medics are, of the terrible toll on human life resulting from 'Spanish flu', inflicted as humanity still reeled from the slaughter of the First World War; but...well; this was the 21st century. We'd had the shock-horror headlines of Ebola, SARS, MERS, bird-flu and, in the UK at least, had survived these without the virus ever coming remotely close to securing a foothold on these shores. This odd sounding bat-derived coronavirus would probably be just another here-today-gone-tomorrow health scare, wouldn't it?

And then the news items from China started to grow in both frightening figures and column-inches, as well as moving up towards the lead news item. Thousands were becoming infected and dying, and it wasn't just the old and frail. The tipping point for me was seeing the picture of Dr Li Wenliyang, the young Chinese ophthalmic surgeon who initially spotted the problem and alerted the authorities, only to be first ignored and later condemned for alarmist comments. Publishing a selfie of himself wearing an oxygen mask and clearly deteriorating under the onslaught of the virus, within days of the photograph and in the second week of February 2020, he was dead himself from the disease.

Castigated by the authorities and accused of *scaremongering*, there can be few occasions where a whistleblower has been more prescient, or paid a higher price in the process of flagging up an emerging public health catastrophe. He showed the most enormous courage.

By late February it was clear that a major global pandemic was upon us. This time, unlike SARS, MERS and Ebola, it wasn't going to pass us by.

My family had a difficult choice. I'd barely seen home since Christmas, what with squally winter weather, storm cancellations, rough seas and the distinctly unattractive prospect of a rough 3½ hour Saturday crossing home on the *Ben My Chree*, followed by a similarly unappealing return trip the following day. Much easier (not least on my stomach) to hunker down in the flat and listen to the wind and rain lashing the slates, rather than braving the Irish Sea in winter gales. However, there was a solitary opportunity in early spring to fly down to South East England and meet up with the family there.

Glenda, my mother-in-law had been sadly widowed in 1999 whilst I'd still been completing my training down in London. Striking up a new relationship with Norman, he had become a close and well-loved member of the family, and a kind of surrogate grandfather to our boys, especially after the loss of my father too, just before Christmas 2010.

Finally succumbing in late 2019 at an impressive age of 95 and after what he himself would have readily acknowledged was an outstanding innings, we had all been invited to a celebration of Norman's life in Eastbourne on the weekend of 14th March 2020. As the number of UK COVID-19 cases grew, so did our trepidation about the planned trip. Looking back, we should have cancelled, but none of us had the slightest idea of the terrible times that lay ahead.

I'd also been invited, via Ed, our oldest son, to deliver a lecture that same weekend to the University College of London Surgical Society on both surgical whistleblowing and urological surgery.

I could double-up, deliver the lecture on the Friday evening and then meet up with the rest of the family in Eastbourne. In the end, we decided to take the plunge.

Flying down to Stanstead, I met up with Ed at Euston and we set about getting ready for the lecture, having the dubious honour of giving the very last, Friday evening, face-to-face UCL lecture before the teaching schedule was closed, everyone was sent home and all lectures cancelled in the face of the oncoming pandemic. It was, however, really wonderful to be back in London again after all those years and in front of a keen, sharp, young and curious surgical audience. I thoroughly enjoyed the experience, relieving memories of my own medical studentship at Charing Cross and Westminster and presentations from my earlier life there. Taking the train to Eastbourne later that evening, we joined up happily with the rest of the family and made straight for Wetherspoons.

Norman's life celebration was worth every effort of getting down there. He'd enjoyed a truly remarkable life, including training with the RAF in the closing months of the second world war. After a distinguished career with Unilever, he'd enjoyed a quantity and quality of retirement that most of us can only dream of.

Here was someone who had had the courage to join up and who was prepared to risk and, possibly, sacrifice their life to fight the Nazi nightmare vision of a totalitarian Europe. There are, as mentioned in *Whistle in the Wind*, so very few of such characters left and, even looking back over the risks that we took by joining with Norman's family for the tribute to his remarkable life, I'm so glad that we made the effort.

Saying our thanks and goodbyes, possibly the last time that we'd get to see Norman's family, the five of us and Glenda took ourselves off for some fresh air over the Seven Sisters on the channel coast. Pulling over into the roadside car park for a short walk, to reflect on our loss and to admire the view over the sea and chalk cliffs, a snarling, urgent, hair-raising and insistent large-petrol-engine note started to make itself known.

What on earth is that? Twisting around over my shoulder as we all got out of the car, I could see no sign of the vehicle in question. *Ferrari? Aston-Martin?* Whatever it was, it sounded like it was being driven at a highly illegal speed.

Then it dawned on me that it was coming from above....

As though paying tribute to one of the very last of the gallant young airmen of 39-45, those who were prepared to fight and risk their lives for their country and their principles, a lone Supermarine Spitfire looped and rolled above the white cliffs, revelling and exulting in the space, light and freedom of the skies, the early-spring sunlight flashing off its wings and the sonorous exhaust seeming to make the very tarmac itself tremble in submission. A sight that must have inspired a young Norman himself, so many times, and so very close to here too, some 75 years ago.

It was a moment of considerable emotion for all of us, as we stood, moist-eyed, watching and listening to this supreme reminder and memory of wartime courage, principles and heroism as it tumbled, spun and weaved through the clouds in what seemed like a dance of life and joy above us.

Norman himself could have wished for no better tribute and send off.

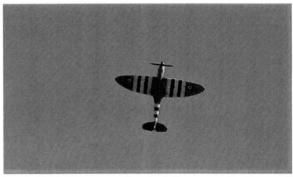

14th March 2020. Supermarine Spitfire over the Seven Sisters.

EASTBOURNE SEEMED GRIPPED BY FEAR and adrenaline that Saturday evening. Lockdown was imminent; I think that we all subconsciously guessed what might be heading towards us. The little Italian restaurant where we ate that evening was otherwise almost entirely empty.

Wetherspoons, however, was heaving. Fiona and Glenda with feminine common sense had decided to have an early night, but Ed, Rob, Will and I, with typical masculine overconfidence, thought we'd have a last drink in honour of Norman. Packed out, with standing room only and, never having had much of a bar-presence, it took me nearly 20 minutes just to get served, only for us to have to bellow in each other's ears, such was the noise of everyone shouting and coughing over everyone else. With much boisterous laughter and banter from all around us, beers being spilled and more of them poured, it was great to have a good family chat and gossip over a few drinks.

Little did we know that, in early 2020, over that very weekend and along with the rest of the UK, this would be our very last trip to a packed pub for a conventional few pints for a very, very long time indeed.

My route back to the Isle of Man was via Gatwick and easyJet. Dropped off the following morning by the rest of the family on their way back to Lancaster, I watched the green fields and villages of South East England fade away through the cloud base, wondering when I might next get to see England, Fiona and the boys again. Increasingly feeling like some kind of displaced, wandering vagrant without any definitive home or base, I consoled myself with the thought that I'd be back in Lancaster very shortly. Two or three weeks at the very most...?

Even at my most pessimistic, I'd never have guessed that it might be mid-August, nearly six months on. Swooping in over the Irish Sea, with the green hills and the beautiful cliffs and rocky panorama of the eastern coast of the Isle of Man opening up beneath us, we were accompanied all the way by the soundtrack of wheezing, hacking dry coughs up and down the aircraft.

Arriving on one of the last few flights in before the Island locked down and closed its borders, I fired up my trusty old BMW and trundled back to Peel, oblivious to the fellow passengers making their way out of the airport and flagging down taxis outside Ballasalla Airport. Only much later was I to hear that at least one of those Manx taxi drivers contracted a fatal dose of COVID-19 from a passenger on those very last flights in.

The Isle of Man locked down just days later at roughly the same time as the rest of the UK. And of course, one of the very first things to get cancelled was regular 'elective' surgery and clinics. At a loose end once I had cleared my outstanding paperwork, it seemed appropriate to volunteer to help out with the Island's COVID response and I found myself spending an enjoyable, if busy number of days donning a headset and helping to man the COVID111 help-lines, deciding who could be reassured, who ought to be self-isolating and who should be reporting to the TT grandstand for swab testing. However, as the swift lockdown started to take effect and overall numbers of new diagnoses stabilised, the pressures soon switched to hospital care.

The Manx population is approximately 85,000, with a fair number of elderly and high-risk patients amongst them. Noble's Hospital is a relatively small hospital with an ICU facility of only six beds. It didn't take much mathematical ability to work out that if only a very small percentage of the population became seriously ill then ICU would be completely overwhelmed. And we couldn't, as we'd normally do, rely on Liverpool to take any overspill. They had their own problems to deal with.

To their great credit, Noble's management and clinicians brought in changes at a remarkably rapid rate. Theatre recovery was closed, every available ventilator commandeered and the area transformed into an impromptu back-up ICU, with theatres themselves cut in two and sealed off, creating a small remaining number of theatres for emergency cases and recovery, and the rest of theatres reconfigured to provide further COVID positive ICU space.

Thankfully, the Manx lockdown and border closures were just about in the nick of time. Noble's was able to cope, but it was very close-run and, with hindsight, another week or two of free travel to and from the island might well have resulted in the hospital being overwhelmed. As it was, the virus rapidly overcame one of the larger nursing homes on the island, ending the lives of 20 residents and rendering many of the staff seriously ill.

Urological surgery, along with all other non-emergency operations took a back seat in these unprecedented times, with all face-to-face clinic appointments being cancelled too. With no end to the lockdown in sight, it seemed sensible to occupy the spare time by going back through our outstanding outpatient referrals.

At the beginning of the lockdown in spring we had a frankly unsatisfactory wait for routine clinic appointments of some 18 to 20 months. Julie, our super-organised urology secretary, produced a good number of heavy lever-arch files full of referrals, and, when I would otherwise have been operating or carrying out clinics or endoscopy lists, I instead began to work through them, writing to anyone where I felt that their problems could be managed in the community, making suggestions, reassuring, organising more tests in the community and writing with prescriptions that they could work through with their GP; telephoning any others where I needed more information. With only urgent or emergency operating lists or endoscopy sessions and with the new referrals coming in being dramatically reduced in number, there was plenty of time to get to work on the outstanding outpatients, and the heavy files of referrals began getting noticeably lighter. With a colossal effort from Julie, hundreds of letters being typed per week and other secretaries drafted in from the secretarial pool, despite the ongoing lockdown we saw our waiting times drop to twelve, then six and, by the end of the crisis in summer, to just a month or two. Whilst the same cannot be said of our waits for surgery, we must be one of the very few units to be coming out of the other end of the pandemic with outpatient clinic waiting times that have been slashed.

As happens with COVID-19, the community cases of transmission were the first to come under control, dwindling away as early summer came on and the Manx local lockdown began to lift in around June. However, the fallout for the hospital continued for some time later, with seriously ill patients remaining on NIV (non-invasive ventilation) or on the ICU for some time after the community cases came under control.

Having got our outpatients under control and with regular operating still cancelled, helping out on the wards seemed to be the correct and appropriate thing to do. Down at University College Medical School in London, Ed was coming to the same conclusions, volunteering, on top of his daytime medical student work, to work nights in ICU and the COVID sections of the Emergency Department at the Royal Free Hospital.

Along with a number of other Noble's Hospital staff volunteers, we all underwent a crash course in non-invasive ventilation, masks, oxygen saturations, ventilators, blood gases, inotropes and the minute-by-minute monitoring of critically ill, ventilated patients. Mercifully, the COVID positive patients never spilled out of Noble's ICU (although it was completely full at one point) and thankfully it never became necessary to use non-ICU staff like myself for essential critical care purposes on the Isle of Man.

Nevertheless, twice a day we had an 'all-hands-on-deck' event for 'proning' the ventilated patients.

This is the technique of nursing COVID patients face down, which improves the lung function and increases oxygen absorption. The technique is well established as a way of optimising the respiratory performance of patients with certain breathing problems, but, to the general public and non-respiratory clinicians like myself, it was pretty much unknown before the outbreak of the COVID-19 pandemic. Much of the standard management of COVID patients from those early days of 2020 has been discarded or superseded now, but 'proning' has survived, particularly for those patients unable to maintain their oxygen levels when supine (on their backs).

However, it isn't possible to manage patients entirely face down. At least twice a day they need to be turned, cleaned, changed and their pressure areas checked and dressed to try and avoid pressure sores and skin breakdown, not least over the patients' faces when they are lying face-down for a significant part of every 24-hour period.

Turning an anaesthetised patient over is fraught with danger and difficulty as, of course, the patient is floppy, completely unconscious and intubated (a tube inserted into the windpipe and connected to the ventilator, essential to keep the patient oxygenated and alive). Also, as in most ICU scenarios, the patients who are intubated for

COVID are a mass of tubes and monitoring equipment, with central lines, arterial lines, catheters, feeding tubes, oxygen saturation monitors, multiple heart monitoring leads etc. Turning everything over in patients often weighing over 100kg without dislodging some vital tube or monitoring equipment or injuring the patient in the process is challenging and hazardous in the extreme, especially when the staff are all wrapped up and anonymised in PPE, their speech and hearing impaired as a consequence of the FFP3 virus proof masks and visors.

The technique itself has seemingly changed little since it was first advised in COVID cases by the Chinese intensivists in early 2020. Slippery slide sheets are inserted beneath the patient so that the patient can slide back and forth easily on the bed. The patient is part-rolled back and forth, with the anaesthetist or one of the experienced ICU staff monitoring the airway, and fresh, clean sheets are placed beneath and on top of the patient, together with fresh pillows if the patient is going face-down in order to protect any bony 'pressure areas' over the hips and chest. With the patient and pillows at the centre of a sandwich of two sheets, a team of seven people readies themselves and a check list is read out to ensure that everything vital is secured and taken care of, and everyone knows their role. Three staff attend to each side of the patient and the most senior anaesthetist controls the airway at the patient's head end. The edges of the top and bottom sheets are rolled up together snugly on both sides, making sure that the patient's arms are by their side, palms facing in, so that the patient and any pillows are wrapped tight between the sheets, forming the shape known to ICU staff as the 'Cornish pasty'. With slide sheets under the patient, with the anaesthetist in charge and controlling the airway and with the six assistants gripping the rolled-up sides of the sheets, the patient is slid sideways to the edge of the bed, then in two more swift movements and with the anaesthetist controlling the whole manoeuvre, up on to their side and then over onto their face, the assistants changing their grip half-way through the manoeuvre. The process is then repeated in reverse some 12 to 18 hours later to turn the patient onto their back again.

It is a tiring and stressful process. Intubated and ventilated patients start to lose muscle mass and bone strength pretty much as soon as they are sedated and ventilated. Particularly after a good number of days of paralysis and mechanical ventilation, it's all too easy for a patient to suffer inadvertent neck or limb injuries when being repeatedly turned back and forth. And, of course, losing control of the airway could be fatal within seconds.

It isn't just risky for the patients. Staff, of course, can be injured and exposed to significant risk despite the provision of PPE and all the other precautions. Several of us got scratched or bitten by infected and disorientated patients during the crisis and, clumsily, at one point I managed to gash my forearm on the sharp, machined metal edge of a well-used ICU COVID clinical waste bin. The cut was relatively minor, but the alcogel that I immediately applied had me instantly weeping into my PPE and blinking through streaming eyes for a good while after. Each staff injury is, of course, followed by days of worry about whether the exposed worker has managed to infect themselves.

Whilst, as far as I recall, we never had more than three or four patients requiring proning at any one time, some of the bigger UK hospitals had many dozens, with specialist proning teams doing little else other than working their way endlessly round the patients, carrying out what must have been like the ICU equivalent of painting the Forth Bridge.

Perhaps the most stressful part of ICU care for the ventilated COVID patient is putting them on the ventilator in the first place. As above, an 'ET tube' (endotracheal tube, to go into the mouth and down the trachea – the main wind pipe) needs to be inserted to enable the ventilator to mechanically shift oxygen back and forth into the lungs. However, to correctly insert this requires the patient to be sedated and paralysed. And, of course, in those critical seconds between the induction of anaesthesia (when the sedating and paralysing drugs start to work) and the ET tube placement and connection to the ventilator (intubation), the patient stops breathing altogether.

Normally, this simply isn't a problem, as the patient can be 'pre-oxygenated' and maybe 10 to 20 seconds without breathing isn't an issue. But when the patient is already on high percentages of oxygen and is still struggling to breathe and is already critically short of oxygen because their lungs are full of inflammation and fluid, those few seconds can be both critical and terrifying.

Oxygen levels in the patient's circulation are typically monitored continuously as *oxygen saturations*. The device for making these measures can often be seen on the patient's finger or earlobe, with a red light shining inside it when taken off. Most patients run an oxygen saturation of close to or up to 100%. Anything less than 95% in a 'normal' patient would cause some concern. With the lung injuries seen in COVID-19, the aim was to accept a degree of *desaturation* and run the patients at 88-92% saturations. As a general rule of thumb, anything less than this would require urgent attention. Anything less than 80% would be cause for great concern. During those awful days, it wasn't unusual to see such patients during the intubation process dropping their oxygen saturations to 75, 70 or even 65%, levels that simply cannot be sustained for any length of time without the serious risk of brain injury or death from lack of oxygen.

Just watching such a process used to leave my heart in my mouth. The very act of intubation can release large amount of the virus into the air, and I have only the most enormous admiration for my anaesthetic friends and colleagues, carrying out such incredibly stressful processes, at significant risk to themselves, under huge pressure and simultaneously having to cope with unfamiliar PPE, masks, visors etc. I simply cannot begin to imagine the toll inflicted on the busier units around the world, where ICU staff have had to cope with over a year of such experiences, with many of the patients that they cared for and formed a bond with, often over many weeks, going on to die without relatives present and without ever regaining consciousness.

———————

AS OUR OWN LOCAL COVID tragedies played out, and the island's lockdown thankfully started to squeeze the life out of the pandemic locally, there was one more disaster to unfold.

Abbotswood Nursing Home is a large, roughly 60 bedded unit on the island, and in mid-April the virus found its way into the home.

As happened in so many other elderly care and nursing homes across the world, the coronavirus wreaked havoc. Some 20 patients died, a good number of staff became seriously unwell, and the surviving patients had to be rapidly evacuated.

But where to? Many of them had tested positive for the virus, and they'd all been exposed to it. So they couldn't be put into other homes or a non-COVID hospital ward without potentially spreading the contagion. And this wasn't something that could be delayed. Decisions needed to be made in the 'here-and-now'.

Once again, the Manx authorities moved remarkably swiftly and came up with an excellent stop-gap solution.

Ward 20, or Newlands, as it was otherwise known, was an old, obsolete and mothballed unit; detached and set away from other buildings in the grounds of Noble's Hospital. Dusty, damp, disused and unloved for a good number of years, it was, within what seemed like just a couple of days, comprehensively stripped out, redecorated and re-equipped with amongst other things, oxygen and suction piped to every bed-head, with a team of nursing staff simply thrown together to try and do their best with the desperately sick and frail survivors of the outbreak.

Normally, the Ward 20 basic structure, equipment and facilities would never have passed health-and-safety rules in a million years, nor would staff have simply been asked to hurl themselves in at the clinical-deep-end and just do their best, but this was almost a kind of war-time spirit of just doing your best with what you could. It was impossible to imagine a more diverse team, with hospital and community nurses, social workers, students, occupational therapists, dieticians, junior doctors, pharmacists, consultants, podiatrists, physiotherapists, porters etc. all just chipping in and doing what they could for these desperately ill patients. Incredibly, especially under such distressing, extraordinary and stressful circumstances, this entire and very stretched team seemed to gel and form a cohesive unit within hours. And for a good number of weeks, 24 hours a day and seven days a week, ward 20, for so long silent, dark, cold and deserted, once again rang to the bustle and clatter of drug rounds, meals being served, staff and patient banter and gossip, beds being changed and pressure areas attended to.

Mealtimes are always a particularly intense point in the 24 hour cycle of an acute care ward. Offering, in my newly spare weekday time to try and help out with feeding, cleaning, clearing up and basic ward jobs, it rapidly became a pleasure rather than a chore, to the point where I'd very happily make my way in for weekends or bank holidays if staffing levels were short.

Passing up through the medical and surgical hierarchy provides a good number of privileges, but there can be no doubt that it also distances you from the day-to-day existence, needs and routines of long-stay patients. It was clear to me during those intense but immensely satisfying weeks just how much the patients gained from the simple human touch and basic acts of compassion. Settling down at breakfast or lunchtime with a needy, frail and disabled patient, a bowl of thickened food and a spoon actually became one of the most rewarding parts of the working day, feeling part of the team and watching all the other patients benefiting from the care and compassion around me. It really was a most intense and immense privilege to work alongside those committed and dedicated Manx nursing staff, and it changed me indelibly and, unlike almost all the other events of the last two years, very much for the better.

It would be neither appropriate nor professional to divulge too much detail, particularly where it might reveal a patient's identity, but I need to try and impart some of the sense of achievement that came out of those desperate weeks.

One particular resident comes to mind. From the fragmentary memories that we gleaned from her, she'd clearly been a keen naturalist in her younger years but had eventually been admitted to Abbotswood Nursing Home in her last few years with frailty and dementia. Even more frail when she arrived on ward 20, she had struggled through and survived the outbreak that had claimed so many other residents but was clearly in a desperately bad way. Seeing her for the first time, with unkempt, long straggly hair, stained nightie, long and untrimmed finger nails, unhealthy looking pressure areas and appearing emaciated; indeed, almost skeletal, bed-bound and seemingly terminally unwell, I wondered just how many hours she still had to live. And as I went off duty that evening, I silently speculated about whether she'd even be there in the morning.

Yet, just a few weeks later, after intensive nursing, physiotherapy, feeding and, perhaps most of all, encouragement, patience, interest and love from staff of all backgrounds, I still have the most intense image of her. Looking at least 10 years younger; well-fed and content, sitting by the open French windows enjoying the sun, and with neatly trimmed, blonde hair blowing back in the warm summer breeze, watching a David Attenborough documentary on a donated iPad, exclaiming, pointing out and naming many of the exotic species in the documentary to the nurse sitting with her. It was a poignant and deeply moving moment, especially when recalling the desperately sick, distressed, disorientated and frail old lady that we had admitted just weeks earlier.

It is a great tribute to those who worked on, and who put together the staff team for ward 20 that, whilst a small number of patients died of old age and frailty on that ward, none of them passed away in distress, pain or indignity, or without at least one member of staff there to attend to them, keep them company and hold their hand.

And not a single one of them died of COVID-19.

And it seems quite right and correct that a disused, neglected and forgotten ward, brought back to life to provide relief to so many elderly patients suffering from the ravages of COVID should, after the outbreak had been tamed, now, in early 2021 be put to use to try and prevent further loss of life from this terrible pandemic.

Ward 20 is now humming with more activity as one of the key COVID-19 vaccination hubs for the Isle of Man.

CHAPTER TWELVE

New Evidence

AFTER THE DISORIENTATING MONTHS of late winter, spring and summer of 2020 and having been prevented from travelling, just like everyone else on the Island, it was a relief to be finally granted special permission by the Manx Government to take a fortnight of compassionate leave to see my family. With England still in the stranglehold of the COVID-19 pandemic and with the Isle of Man, at least for the moment having beaten the virus and seeming COVID free; going home was perhaps the most deeply disorientating experience so far. Back on the Isle of Man and at Noble's Hospital, life had returned to normal. But in Lancaster, which I hadn't seen in over six months, it was anything but. Eschewing contact with anyone but immediate family, we cancelled our planned Sicilian holiday and simply agreed to spend a precious two weeks at home, in a house that, unsettlingly, felt like one that I'd moved out of many years ago.

The climate in Northern Lancashire is far from guaranteed, even in August, but fortunately the weather-gods smiled on us and we enjoyed a wonderful fortnight of local walks, barbecues and family nights in with the television and Netflix. Having had no family time together since Christmas 2019 and the subsequent Eastbourne trip, I headed back to the Isle of Man with a good tan, happy memories, a few extra pounds, a sunburned bald-patch and a sense of trepidation. With the Isle of Man COVID free, not only did I have to go into self-isolation for a fortnight on my return, but I had my first interview with Niche Consulting (the NHS England-appointed investigators) coming up and, most importantly, as the weather began to cool, the darker nights closed in and COVID numbers in England almost inevitably began to twitch up again, it now seemed unlikely that we'd be together again as a family until Christmas at the earliest.

Standing on the stern of the *Ben My Chree* as she steamed out of Heysham Port, looking regretfully back over Heysham, Lancaster and the sunlit Bowland Fells, Yorkshire to the east, and the beautiful Lake District to the north, I gave little more than a fleeting thought to my forthcoming interview with Niche. I'd gone through this depressing leaving home torture so very many times over the previous four years, and it never got any easier – attempting to stoically and impassively watch the rolling hills and mountains of Cumbria and Lancashire fade away into the sea haze and the far distance, whilst screaming internally and silently lamenting the family life that, just like hundreds of times before, I was being forced to leave behind.

On that late August Sunday afternoon, I barely thought of Niche. I was far more preoccupied with how I'd cope psychologically after leaving a house that, in the last few days, had actually started to feel like home again, and returning back to my rented flat, two weeks of self-isolation, and an unknown period of time before I'd get to see family and friends once more. My previous face-to-face informal meeting with the NHS England investigators had been low key, friendly and sympathetic and I had no reason to believe that the next *Teams* meeting that they'd requested would be anything different.

How very very wrong I was proved to be.

As with most jobs, I was faced with a mountain of paperwork on my return and, compelled for my first two weeks back to wear PPE at all times except when in my flat and without being able to get out for any outdoor exercise or fresh air,[6] it was already a very depressing start to September 2020 indeed. On the morning of the 11th September, I logged on to Microsoft Teams, pushing to one side the mountain of outstanding paperwork and results, all jostling for my attention, and turned my thoughts to the forthcoming interview, being conducted by the Niche team of Mary-Ann Bruce and Phil

---

[6] Like some other returning Manx healthcare workers, I was allowed to go to work as long as PPE was worn at all times. At all other times and if not working, I was obliged to self-isolate alone in my flat.

Cornford, honorary professor of urology at the Royal Liverpool and Broadgreen NHS Trust.

The exchanges began relatively easily and amicably, with general outlines, rules and pleasantries. However, the questioning quickly began to develop a sharper edge as we homed in on the 'Patient A' Peter Read case. I was told that I hadn't actually formally documented the fact that, when carrying out a check cystoscopy (bladder inspection) and stent change on Peter Read in early 2014, I'd found no sign of any residual bladder cancer. Shrugging, I pointed out that if the procedure had gone straightforwardly, the operation notes reflected this and I hadn't recorded any bladder tumour then, very clearly, I hadn't found any and there wasn't any to record.

In my defence, our operating lists at this time were under significant pressure, with a fast turnover from a slick anaesthetic team and to keep the pace up I'd instinctively turned to minimising the laborious typing out of operative notes, discharge summaries, TTO (To Take Out) medication orders and phone calls or emails to Alison Birtle in the oncology department, or Rachel in the waiting list office regarding follow up. All too often, attempts to meticulously tap out and print off every last detail of the case, particularly with sluggish and sometimes crashing or frozen software, would end up with the next anaesthetised case being wheeled into theatre long before I'd finished all of the above jobs, with the distinct possibility that they'd then not get done at all, or only after the list was over, with the risk of confusing the different patients on that particular operating list.

Quietly making a mental note to learn and improve from this, make my note taking at Noble's Hospital a little more voluminous and document the things that I hadn't found or done, as well as the positives and technicalities, the heat was suddenly turned up a lot further...

...OK. The 26ᵗʰ December 2014 Mr Duffy.... The on-call general surgical team phone you up and say what to you...?

Oh no...no...no...no.... Please no.... For Heaven's sake! Surely not this again?? How many more times?

I just couldn't believe that, once more, we were back, all over again, to this particular piece of historical fiction. I and Peter Read's family had repeatedly and consistently rejected this false allegation and implication, over and over again, dating all the way back to the discredited statements made in 2015. To his credit, Ian Pearce's final draft of the RCA had made it clear that there was not the slightest shred of evidence in support of an emergency general surgical referral to me that day, either formal or informal. Yet, here we were, despite Ian's conclusions and the family's testimony, regressing five years with yet another brazen attempt to try and force feed this nasty little bit of fiction to me again, shift the point of the first missed opportunity back 24 to 48 hours and manipulate me into accepting responsibility for the first clinical error in Peter Read's death.

It suddenly felt like I was back under hostile cross-examination once again. Back in the employment tribunal or the GMC's hearing of 2019, and into yet another *double jeopardy* situation with, once more, tricky attempts to try and manipulate my responses in such a way as to lead me into self-incrimination. Except this time, I realised to my horror, I didn't have any legal or impartial representation to keep things fair and appropriate.

Pointing out nervously, yet once again, that there had never been a general surgical referral, I couldn't help but reflect on just how many attempts had been made to try and either wear me down or ram this particular falsehood down my throat. There never was the slightest hint of any emergency situation or sepsis on 26th December 2014 and never, at any point, had I picked up any sense, either from the family or the nurses, of any incipient or concurrent major deterioration, simply a commonsense desire from the family and ward staff to at least discuss bringing forward one aspect of Peter Read's care that had already been deferred, namely his regular, planned urological stent change.

I spelled out to Niche how the exchange with the family had gone, comparing it with the kind of exchange of information that might go on if I had taken a call in the office from an anxious family, keen to speak to the consultant about expediting a relative's procedure. In other words, low-key, hopefully sympathetic, business-like and obliging. I pointed out that I had then gone on to explain the new plan to Mr Read himself, sitting by his bedside and making sure that he was clear and happy about the plan for the stent change to go ahead on the following Monday afternoon or Tuesday if he was still in hospital.

Distracted by the sudden realisation that this had turned into a far more hostile and dangerous process than I'd been led to believe, I still wasn't paying full attention when the next question landed.

Mr Duffy, can we take you back to the email you sent to the waiting list office on that day, December 26th 2014?

Well…this was going to be difficult. There was no doubt that an email had been sent. I'd told the family that I'd send it, we'd agreed on surgery on the Monday afternoon on Carl Rowbotham's operating list, or alternatively my own Tuesday list, and, after all, it was documented in the notes. And I would have sent it to Rachel Minshull, my regular contact in the waiting list office, possibly copying Carl in. But of course, nearly six years on, I couldn't remember the exact contents.

Mary-Ann read the email out to me. It was dated the 26th, sent to the waiting list office by myself and referred to Peter Read by name and hospital number. It sounded vaguely authentic, but thinking through the contents, little bits didn't add up.

Why would I have sent it to both Heidi and Angela, and not to Rachel? That's odd….. I'd always automatically contact Rachel, as she was the default urology person in the waiting list office. Why would I have left her out? And why would I have copied the email to (consultant A) *and Mr Cutting, especially when all I was doing was to bring forward the date of a routine operation? Why would they need to know? Especially when the list alteration only involved either Mr Rowbotham or myself.*

That just doesn't make any sense at all….

We knocked the content of this email back and forth for a few minutes. I was genuinely puzzled. It didn't seem remotely logical from my point of view, particularly as it referred to Mr Read's stent as being blocked.

How could I possibly have figured that out? Peter Read's creatinine (a blood test measure of kidney function) had taken a huge jump in the early hours of the following morning, some 12 hours after I'd left the ward, thereby screaming out the presence of a new kidney problem and likely stent blockage. However, the latest results available to me on the 26th from the previous day (the 25th – Christmas Day) had been essentially normal. The big deterioration in Mr Read's kidney function was the following day (the 27th). And I didn't even recall looking any blood results up. Why on earth would I have? All I had done was to informally pop into the ward at the request of the staff to speak to the family. There was no reason why I'd be checking on blood results or speculating on a possible stent blockage to the waiting list office, especially when there was no evidence to suggest such an event.

And I'd also implied that Mr Read was deteriorating and that he wouldn't be fit for emergency surgery over the weekend. That was just plain wrong. The general surgeons, according to the notes, had been discharge planning that morning and clearly thought that Peter might soon be in a position to go home. Why on earth would I have then claimed that he wasn't fit enough for theatre over the weekend? I hadn't done any kind of assessment of his fitness for theatre, and neither had anyone else. Nor was there any indication for an anaesthetic assessment. No one was remotely considering emergency urological surgery at that point anyway. And I had gone on to suggest that Peter was therefore booked for theatre the following week implying that, although he'd be too unfit to have emergency surgery over the weekend, somehow Mr Read would have miraculously recovered his fitness sufficiently for theatre after the weekend was over. So much so, in fact, that by then he'd be fit for a regular *elective* procedure.

That was complete rubbish too....

Our anaesthetic colleagues willingly anaesthetise unfit patients in an emergency scenario if urgent or life-saving surgery is required, but would have no hesitation in cancelling an unfit, high-anaesthetic-risk patient who had been listed for routine surgery. And if Mr Read was unfit for emergency anaesthesia and surgery over the weekend – and was deteriorating too, then it was cast-iron guaranteed that he'd be turned down for elective surgery the following week.

And I'd booked Mr Read for theatre for the following Monday or Tuesday after bumping into Peter's family on my way into the ward. The assurance that I'd book Peter for the next week had been made to his family there and then. It was simply a logical decision and had nothing to do with Peter's anaesthetic fitness or lack of it. Why on earth would I have worked such a silly and contradictory statement about anaesthetic risks and unsuitability for emergency surgery into the email when all I was doing was expediting a planned, routine procedure?

The whole thrust of my email was incoherent and contradictory....

However, my puzzlement and head-scratching were obliterated within an instant. It was, I later confessed, like having an anvil dropped out of a clear blue sky on to me.

Mr Duffy, do you recall what you were doing on Monday the 29th December? No? Well, you were doing an extra clinic at the Queen Victoria Hospital in Morecambe. You remember that? No? OK, well, that is where you were. You'd spent the morning doing administrative work with your secretary and were in clinic in Morecambe that afternoon.

Wondering where this was going, I was asked.... *You were on-call that evening?*

Yes, was the answer. I remembered the exchanges in the RCA meeting with Ian Pearce. Consultant B, my on-call ex-colleague for the 29th had argued the case for the Monday being a bank holiday and had tried to imply that, as a consequence, it wasn't his responsibility to hand Peter Read over that evening. We'd all rejected this, agreeing that it certainly was not a bank holiday and that there had been no handover, but no one could recall who was on call that evening. However, by the time of the video-linked M&M meeting, it had emerged that it was me.

Talking this through, I made it clear to Phil and Mary-Ann that, had Peter Read been handed over to me that evening, then, bearing in mind his clear and acute deterioration over the previous 60 hours or so, I'd have had him in theatre just as quickly as it could possibly be arranged.

Peter, we have an email sent from you at approximately 4pm. Do you remember a telephone conversation with Dr Highley – from ICU?

I didn't remember any such thing.

Mr R has indeed gone off big time and is now on the ICU on an adrenaline infusion. Mary-Ann read out to me.
Just had Dave Highley, ICU consultant, on the phone asking if I can change the stent either tonight or tomorrow. Will go and assess after the clinic. Please could he be provisionally added to tomorrow's list in case I can't do him tonight. Thanks very much.

It was as though something had exploded inside my head.
The pain was just utterly, utterly unbearable.
*Oh my dear, sweet God...*where on earth had all this new information come from, and how could I possibly have taken such a phone call, tapped out this email and then simply turned back to my clinic and completely forgotten about such a critically ill patient?
The point was driven home utterly mercilessly to me. Each additional fact was like someone hammering another nail into my already screaming head.

You've attached the email from the 26th to this one from the 29th and addressed it to Heidi and Angela saying that you'll review the patient after clinic....
No, in answer to your question, there's nothing recorded in the ICU notes about this phone call, about you reviewing Peter Read or getting him to theatre that evening.

Left reeling from this revelation, all I could blurt out was my shock and disbelief.... And....

Are you sure this is genuine?!

Mary-Ann and Phil were absolutely clear that they thought the email to be genuine. *You sent it to Heidi and Angela and copied it to Colin Cutting, as well as (Mr A) and (Mr B). Why would you do that?*

Now, you took over the on-call responsibility at 6 o'clock? Yes? You carried out an emergency testicular torsion operation that evening.... Do you remember? No? Well, you did. At about 8pm.

No Peter, we can confirm that no one responded to, actioned or acknowledged this email, or indeed the one from the 26th. Can you explain any of this?

Of course, I couldn't. The whole thing made no sense whatsoever. Why would I have received such a call at 4pm about an emergency case when I wasn't on-call until 6 o clock, and indeed wasn't even in Lancaster? UHMBT switchboard had a copy of the on-call rota and would have automatically put any urgent calls through to the on-call urological surgeon. And why would I have accepted responsibility for the patient when I was on the opposite side of Lancaster and Morecambe, at least 30 minutes' drive away and half-way through a clinic when there was someone on site at Lancaster precisely to deal with exactly this kind of immediate emergency? Someone who had already reviewed the patient earlier that day and was much more up to date with what was going on.

And, if such a call had taken place and I had accepted responsibility for the patient, why was I holding up the Morecambe clinic and laboriously writing emails about it, copying them through to two people who were actively looking to cause trouble for me and then forgetting about the case completely, rather than immediately cancelling the rest of the clinic, jumping into the car and heading straight back to Lancaster to deal with the emergency problem?

How on earth had I made such a terrible error of judgement? Yes, I was busy and distracted with other patients and wasn't on-call, so probably wasn't fully alert to emergencies. And perhaps, as Mary-Ann had implied, I'd been distracted on my way back by a call about the possible emergency torsion case. But.... But.... But...?

But if I'd wanted Peter Read listing for the following day, why on earth didn't I just ring the waiting list office and ask them to book it there and then? I'd always do that for an urgent case, and I knew Rachel's number off by heart. It'd have taken thirty seconds, rather than laboriously typing out a complex email, searching for and attaching a previous email and then copying in several people who were not immediately relevant to the emergency, all whilst I was in the middle of a busy clinic and with patients waiting outside. And why, just like the email of the 26th, hadn't I sent it to Rachel, my usual contact in the waiting list office? And if I was going to copy anyone in, surely it would have been Dave Highley? After all, he was the person that I was responding to. And this had been sent to two people, copied to three others in working hours and flagged as *high priority*. How come no one ever replied or acted on it? Or indeed even remembered it?

And surely, if I really had sent this email, I'd assuredly have asked for Peter Read to take priority and go first on the operating list the following day. Yet, the way that the email read, Peter could easily have ended up as the last patient on the list – over 24 hours later.

It simply made no sense whatsoever. And most of all, how could I possibly have calmly turned back to my clinic, methodically worked through it all and then simply headed off back to Lancaster and home, completely forgetting about this critically ill man, in need of immediate surgery?

Trembling, mindful of the anonymous tip-off and disbelieving of whether such explosive and pivotal evidence really could have remained completely concealed and forgotten about since 2014, I again questioned whether the emails seemed to be authentic.

Yes, I was firmly told.

And after all, emails never lie do they, I told myself. *It's not like paper medical or nursing notes that can be tampered with. Where pages or results can get 'lost' or replaced; or where an extra line or two, or a new page can be quietly and anonymously slipped into the clinical record.*

Once an email is sent, well...that's it. Done. It's set in stone....

Mary-Ann held up a paper copy of the email of the 29th with the attached email of the 26th and, although most of the text was not visible, I could get a glimpse of my name in the title.

From:	Duffy Peter (UHMB) <Peter.Duffy@mbht.nhs.uk>
Sent:	29 December 2014 16:02
To:	Mckenzie Heidi (UHMB); Angela Jackson
Cc:	Colin Cutting; ▉▉▉ A ; ▉▉▉▉ B
Subject:	RE: urgent case for tuesday
Importance:	High

Ladies

Mr R has indeed gone off big-time and is now on ICU on adrenaline infusion. Just had Dave Hiley (ICU consultant) on phone asking if I can change stent either tonight or tomorrow. Will go and assess after clinic. Please could he be provisionally added to 2moz list in case I can't do him tonight?

Thanks v much

Peter

From: Duffy Peter (UHMB)
Sent: 26 December 2014 16:55
To: Mckenzie Heidi (UHMB); Jackson Angela (UHMB)
Cc: Cutting Colin (UHMB); ▉ A ▉▉▉ (UHMB)
Subject: urgent case for tuesday

Heidi

Just wondering what you've got on Tuesday? We have Peter Read, RTX▉▉▉ on ward 33 who seems to be deteriorating according to his family. Needs cystoscopy, change of left JJ stent. He's a pt of carl and John who was turned down for surgery earlier this month @ bowel obstruction and has had intermittent abdominal pain and bloating since. Doesn't look fit to be done as an emergency over the weekend, but also has a blocked stent so will need doing sooner rather than later. Is it possible to add him to the list?

Thx

peter

So, there it was. It could only possibly have come from me. Clearly, I'd had the most terrible lapse of clinical standards, memory and integrity. Here was clear, incontestable evidence that I could have got Peter Read to theatre 12 to 15 hours earlier than I did. It was truly, totally and utterly devastating, and, having instinctively acknowledged my clear culpability and neglect to Mary-Ann and Phil, I sat there, dazed, in silence, with my heart racing; numb, trembling and disbelieving at the sheer extent of my hypocrisy and failings.

Just moments earlier, I'd insisted to Mary-Ann and Phil that, had I been informed of Peter Read's predicament, I'd have had him in theatre that evening. And now, within seconds of making that statement, this shattering new evidence had, it seemed, potentially shown me up in the investigator's eyes as a potential liar, fraud, hypocrite and manipulator of evidence.

And, of course, I'd previously compared the events around Peter Read's avoidable death to a well-documented UK gross negligence manslaughter case, which in turn had led to a spell in prison for the erring urological surgeon. And now here I was, having shown the same casual, hands-off attitudes, having flagged up the failings of others and now, as a result of an email from my own hand, being clearly shown up as neglectful and potentially negligent myself.

Was this going to end in a jail sentence?

Maybe that was what I deserved?

After all the other awful things that have happened, I really don't think I could ever possibly face that....

This surely, was the utter ruination of me as a doctor, and the end of any remaining self-respect and self-confidence as a competent clinician and decent human being.

———

THE REST OF THE INTERVIEW passed in a blur. To this day, I have absolutely no idea how I staggered through the desperate hours, days and weeks that followed. With the borders of the Isle of Man locked tightly closed, I couldn't even get back for a Saturday night to find some solace, company and distraction with my family and friends. And at the time of the interview and for several days after, I was still in modified self-isolation anyway, only allowed into the hospital in PPE and not allowed to leave the flat for any other purposes whatsoever.

Having been forced out of my chosen career and vocation in Morecambe Bay, having little choice but to leave behind my much loved family and friends and unwillingly take up a lonely and solitary lifestyle on the Isle of Man, with the family and social separation being dramatically worsened by the COVID lockdown and an increasing sense of being rootless and of *no fixed abode,* about all I had left from four decades of hard graft was my professional commitment, pride and standards.

And now even this last remaining achievement had been comprehensively stripped away from me, with no warning and in what felt like the most horrible, ruthless and brutal possible fashion.

All I could think about was how I'd let myself, my family, my profession and above all else, Peter Read and his family down, and whether I could possibly ever survive a spell in prison.

To make matters even worse still, just a few days later, sitting numbly in front of my office desktop and trying desperately to concentrate on clinical matters, a new email message pinged in, marked *General Medical Council.*

Oh no…. Surely not more bad news…?

It was. The GMC, in addition to my ongoing *fitness to practice* enquiry, were now also in possession of these two previously undiscovered emails.

Did I recognise them and accept ownership of them?

Rather oddly, as well as asking if I recognised the emails, and in response to my reply, the GMC were noticeably reluctant to disclose exactly how, during what was supposed to be a highly secret and confidential NHS England enquiry, such explosive new evidence had ended up almost instantaneously in the hands of the medical regulator.

And where did my responsibilities lie now? Niche on behalf of NHS England were very clearly of the opinion that I should not risk potentially upsetting Peter Read's family with the shock revelation of this new information.

On the other hand, how did this fit with my professional duty of candour, and my personal desire to confess my failings and apologise?

Running through the whole awful and distressing business with Fiona and Edward, our eldest, we quickly agreed that my duty of candour clearly trumped any allegiances that I might have to Niche and NHS England, and I should speak to Mr Read's family.

Phoning Karen, Peter Read's daughter, was the most difficult thing I have ever done. Still confined to my flat in the evenings and weekends as a part of my ongoing self-isolation, I sat in the evening darkness and took her through my terrible failings. Karen listened in silence as I profusely apologised over and over again, and stumbled through my confession to her that, somehow, incredibly, I had diagnosed the presence of a blocked kidney stent in her father on the Friday despite the lack of any up-to-date imaging and despite Peter Read's last creatinine blood test (a measure of kidney function) being normal. Inexplicably, despite such a diagnostic feat, I had failed to act, and had, utterly inexcusably, completely forgotten about his predicament after the telephone alert, late afternoon on the Monday the 29th from Dr Highley on ICU, despite documenting it all in a highly detailed email.

I was braced for an explosion of anger, hate and resentment from Karen. It was, after all, only human to react with fury and rage under such circumstances, especially after what had already happened to her father, and when it might appear that I'd been very selective with the facts.

Karen's reaction couldn't have been more different from my expectations. But in some ways and having already accepted that I fully deserved a very generous dose of abuse, it just made my distress worse.

Well, whatever you did or didn't do on that Friday or Monday, you were still the only person who showed any interest or did anything meaningful to help. And you're the only person to make any kind of meaningful attempt to apologise too, and to help us put together what went on. So, we're not angry with you and we still appreciate the things you tried to do....

And the very last thing we'd want would be for you to do something silly; like resign and hand in your GMC registration over this....

All I recall was being desperately, deeply and inconsolably distressed at this point, to the point where at one stage and for several minutes I couldn't even articulate my words or thoughts. In many ways it would have been so very much easier if Karen had put me on the defensive and ranted and raved about my neglect and inadequacies. Kindness, civility, thoughtfulness and understanding was simply not something that I'd predicted or prepared myself for. Putting down the phone after we'd agreed to speak again soon, I sat, trembling in the gloom, not wanting to turn the lights on in case I caught sight of myself in the mirror, and with just my dark agonies, moist, unfocused eyes, and extreme and utter self-loathing and contempt for company.

I've no idea how long I sat there in the darkness, but it must have been a very long time. Finally, a ping from my mobile made me jump violently. It was a message from Karen. She'd spoken to her family and Nicola, her sister, felt the same. The family hadn't lost confidence in me. They were still grateful for my intervention and were also grateful that I'd been open enough to contact them and apologise for the extent of my own failings in the death of their father.

The Read family's continuing support, despite my newly discovered inadequacies, at least offered me some kind of comfort as I staggered through the blurred and never ending daylight hours and twisted and turned through endless sleepless nights, agonising over my lack of action and clinical failings, whether I myself might now be the subject of a police investigation for manslaughter and whether I should do the immediate, decent, honourable thing and immediately resign my job, registration and medical qualifications over my error.

A second Niche interview and various telephone calls came and went in a similar haze of disbelief and self-doubt, with us going round in circles over these emails. I just couldn't get my head around a clinical error of this magnitude. Repeatedly assured that, from Niche's perspective, the two emails looked perfectly genuine, I was told that the characteristics of these emails didn't fit with my previous requests for information or evidence during the earlier enquiries and tribunal processes, and that was why they'd never come to light before.

The cottage is big and old – very old. And very rambling. Probably several old workmen's cottages knocked into one, with lots of small rooms, all interlinked and with steps up and down, steep cramped stairways, low ceilings to bump your head on, furniture, rugs and carpets to trip over…like some three-dimensional labyrinth, and all in near darkness; just a sliver of silvery moonlight filtering through the occasional small, leaded window.

I'm moving silently from room to room, sensing my way around this unfamiliar maze, running my hands along the rough, whitewashed plaster and feeling in the gloom with each silent footfall for an unexpected step or staircase. I can just about make out the shadowy silhouette of each room as I slip through soundlessly and on to the next.

And all the time, I can sense something following me. A presence; an aura…but when I look fearfully over my shoulder, I can see nothing in the shadows and darkness.

But still I keep moving, and still that spectral presence is there; behind me.

And then I'm in a bedroom, with a large double bed.

And no door out on the other side.

I'm trapped.

I sit down on the bed and sense the presence; a dark and insubstantial apparition, slide in through the darkened door. It's facing me now, back to the wall.

And a glimmering face comes into view; shades of grey, like a darkened camera image slowly coming into focus. I squint, trying to make out the features. And then I'm overjoyed. It is William, our youngest boy. He's reaching out his arms for a hug. I stand and move towards him, my heart full of happiness, reaching out for an embrace….

And just as I'm within reach, William's face begins to slide and move, like liquid mercury or melting wax, and, in a blind, frantic panic, I realise that it's not William at all.

But it's too late. I'm now embraced. The face distorts, and out of the flowing silvery, molten image comes a new face.

A ram's skull, with empty, vacant eye-sockets, rotten teeth and grotesque coiled horns. Mouth opening, it lunges towards me….

And a voice screams into my mind.

'Lucifer…!!!'

And I'm thrashing and tangled in the duvet, screaming and fighting an imaginary figure that's still part there in the darkness. And then the image fades, and I'm lying on sweat soaked sheets, knuckles white and trembling, panting, and my hands still clenched around crumpled pillows.

———————

EARLY THE FOLLOWING WEEK, and after a fortnight of being unable to take any outdoor exercise or leave the flat at all except for work, I was at last allowed out of self-isolation and was free to do some evening shopping and have a walk in the night-time salt-fresh sea air of Peel. It was a dark, cold and deeply gloomy trip out. Half-heartedly collecting some meagre rations from the local supermarket (I lost half a stone in the week that followed these revelations), I dumped them in the fridge before heading out to listlessly prowl the shadowy, dimly lit local streets, endlessly running through the sequence of events on the Friday and Monday of December 2014, like some video on permanent replay.

I desperately needed some company that evening, even just the odd passing stranger, or the sounds of a child's laughter or a scolding parent, but the streets of Peel, normally resonant with the noises and salt smells of a seaside fishing town seemed strangely empty and featureless that evening.

Disorientated with sleeplessness, each darkened alley stretched out to infinity, like some miserable, dim, fearful tunnel reaching out to eternity, and every step seemed leaden, as though the sheer weight and responsibility for my incompetence and neglect was pressing me down into the damp, glistening pavement.

How **could** I have been so casual and careless, I raged at myself? I'd made such a fuss whilst at UHMBT about the need for immediate surgery in cases just like this…. Time and again I'd pointed out the dangers of gambling with lives, knowingly neglecting cases exactly like this and leaving them for someone else to sort out. But here I was, having criticised others, and now being exposed as an utter hypocrite, liar and neglectful doctor myself. Not only had I let down a patient and family, I'd betrayed the standards of my profession, my own family, friends and my speciality.

What a truly, utterly hopeless surgeon I'd turned out to be; a liability and hazard to my patients and a proper disgrace to my profession and my mentors, walking away from and forgetting about a needy and desperately sick man.

Self-loathing turned to deep, focused anger. How could I possibly live with myself after this? And with a possible criminal record too.... How could I ever again face my family, friends and those ex-colleagues who'd so loyally supported me?

I've no idea how far, or for how long I walked that evening, until the distant grinding of gears and clatter of an accelerating diesel engine tripped me out of my distress and introspection. Instinctively squeezing into a narrow, recessed doorway in the alley, I watched over my shoulder as the lights of a large, squat and heavy-looking builder's truck swung ponderously round the end of the ginnel and rapidly picked up speed towards me.

He's giving that engine some stick....

And then the dark and self-destructive impulses of the last few days coalesced and melded together.

It was immediately, abundantly clear how everything could be instantly resolved.

Everything.

The vehicle accelerated towards me, but it seemed, in my mind, to be slowing at the same time. My thoughts snapped into focus. It was a moment, above all, of supreme, crystalline clarity and certainty.

Here was the ultimate way to settle this and to escape from this terrible trap that I'd managed to ensnare myself in. A brief, brilliant, split-second flash of pain; appropriate punishment for my terrible lapse in standards, and then endless, painless, wonderful, blissful sleep. A life for a life. No more self-loathing, remorse, hopelessness, responsibility and miserable self-contempt. No need to torture myself any longer with endless re-runs of my greatest career failure.

No need to burden down or ever face again the families, friends, relatives and colleagues that I'd let down so badly. No public humiliation, GMC investigations, prosecution, more hostile cross-examinations, criminal record and a possible jail sentence.

Better to end it now. A quick clean finish. An instant, definitive, irreversible closing down of what was left of my life, before the state and the legal process did it for me. The unfaceable future forever erased; an eternity of oblivion, and the ultimate act of honour and contrition; perfect solution and release.

It all seemed so utterly correct, logical and alluring.

Beautiful even.

The vehicle, still accelerating, slowed some more, rather like the detailed replay of the precise strike in a slow-motion goal. A new interplay of emotions and sensations presented themselves.

Dawn's winter sunlight on a crystalline, frozen lawn. The soft, fragrant breath of a summer's breeze on a high Lakeland fell. Laughter, play and innocent cuddles from an as-yet unborn grandchild. A fine, chilled wine. Birds singing into a vivid Lancashire sunset. The smell of fresh rain on spring bluebells and wild garlic. The soft-stroked, warm velvety coat of a cat, asleep in the warm summer sunshine. The sunny thrill of a skylark's beautiful song on high, remote Yorkshire moors.

So sad. Did I really want to forever say goodbye to these things...?

And what if I survived, but was left horribly mutilated and injured?

But then again, that so-compelling allure of permanent release and unburdening; nothing but darkness and emptiness, an endless infinity of blank, trouble-free and painless pages.

In that last frozen, eternal instant, I was looking down from above; watching myself, huddled, alone and cowering in a shadowy cottage doorway.

It all seemed so exquisitely balanced....

Smoke and Mirrors

CHAPTER THIRTEEN

Decision

THE SLIPSTREAM FROM THE TRUCK was brutal enough to almost tear the beanie from my head. Squashed into the shadowed doorway in a dark, navy jacket and black woollen hat, I was unsure as to whether the speeding truck driver ever even saw me in the late evening darkness. But, in that last life-long, jumbled, split eternal-second of commitment, cowardice, fear and guilt, I'd seen a new vision.

A broken, horribly mutilated and mangled, torn, crushed and bloodied corpse; unrecognisable, with limbs smashed and askew. Funeral; distraught family and relatives. More lives blighted.

Another avoidable death.

And those inconsistencies....

Niche were clear that the emails appeared genuine. They're highly trained and extremely experienced investigators, after all. And they've put Peter Read's case and the evidence relating to it at the very epicentre of their investigations.... They must've done a huge amount of due diligence on these emails.

...but what if they were wrong? And I'd been deceived into throwing my life away over a lie...?

And Peter Read's family? Karen had been so frightened that I might do something like this. Would they have wanted such an ending?

Knees trembling and wanting to bend the wrong way and swallowing back the hot vomit that had found its way into the back of my throat, I made my wobbly way through a metal barrier, towards a low wall and sank down onto it, head in hands and ignoring the dampness from the wet, gritty concrete.

The clatter and red tail-lights receded into the darkness, leaving only the sour, acrid taste of diesel and bile in the back of my throat.

Dear God…that was a close one….

Shakily, sometime, perhaps a lifetime later, I got up and made my unsteady way back to the flat.

No, I wouldn't – couldn't allow this to destroy me. I wouldn't let those who'd wanted to break, silence and destroy me from the start have that final satisfaction. But how close; how very, very terrifyingly close this latest revelation had come to doing exactly that….

I slept just a little better that night.

After days of depression, anxiety and suicidal, self-destructive impulses, I'd been presented with the perfect opportunity to escape from this terrible corner that I'd finished up in. Mercifully, I'd managed, at the very last split-second, to cling on to a sense of perspective.

I'd carry-on fighting this, and fighting to get the full truth of what had happened out, both for myself, for my own family and for Peter Read's family.

But still the thoughts came.

How COULD I have been so casual and incompetent?

CHAPTER FOURTEEN

Questions

NICHE CONSULTING SEEMED MORE than a little unhappy about me contacting the Read family to apologise about this new evidence, and they made this clear, but at least they acknowledged the importance of being open and honest. There seemed no doubt whatsoever that, according to these new emails, I'd been responsible for a massive lapse in my personal and professional standards.

But still those little nagging doubts plagued me.

If I'd had that call from Dave Highley, the ICU consultant, why did I go to ward 33 to find Peter Read on the Tuesday morning, and not to the Intensive Care Unit, where I'd clearly acknowledged that he had been moved to? Could I really have been <u>that</u> forgetful? Surely not? And, if that phone call really had been made, and I hadn't turned up on ICU that Monday evening as promised, why didn't Dave phone me back and chase me up? We knew each other well enough that he'd not have hesitated to remind me, nor would I ever have taken the slightest offence at being chased. And he'd been on duty and in the unit, attending to Mr Read amongst others until the early hours of Tuesday, and would, if these emails were legitimate, have been waiting for me to turn up and make a decision.

ICU didn't seem, from my recollection of the medical or nursing notes, to have any expectation of theatre that evening, nor was there any attempt to prepare Mr Read for such an intervention. Yet this email suggested a major change of plan for the evening and, if that conversation really had taken place, ICU would have documented this new strategy, informed the Read family and would have been working feverishly with the on-call anaesthetist to optimise Peter in time for what the email implied was the clear aim of emergency surgery, just as soon as I got back to Lancaster from the Morecambe clinic.

And if I'd really spoken to Dave and we'd agreed the management plan laid out in the second email, there would have been two things that I'd surely have asked him to do whilst I quickly wrapped things up at Morecambe and headed back to the RLI.

Firstly, to get some imaging (either a CT scan or ultrasound scan; exactly as happened when I discovered Mr Read's predicament the next morning), not least to check that Peter's other kidney didn't need draining too, and secondly to get him booked on the emergency operating list there and then (just as I'd done on discovering Peter Read's predicament the following morning). It has always been a mantra of mine, wherever a case might need to go for emergency surgery, to book the case immediately. Far easier to book the case, do the background investigative work and imaging and then cancel it if you change your mind. If you don't book ahead, then long and hard experience dictates that you arrive sometime later in the operating theatre, armed with the patient's details and latest results, ready to decisively get on with the case as soon as possible, only to find the emergency list already full of cases of fractures, abscesses, appendicitis and other assorted emergencies that got there before you.

When your own case may need immediate emergency attention, far, far better to book as soon as you hear the first news and get in at the front of the queue. But here, despite the fact that this was an absolutely immediate emergency, Dr Highley was just a few yards from theatre and, as senior anaesthetist and ICU lead, could easily have ensured both emergency imaging and that Mr Read's case went first, according to the way this email portrayed events, we seemingly hadn't even discussed informing radiology or theatres, nor had I phoned and notified theatres of the plan myself despite the fact that I knew the number off by heart.

It didn't add up at all.

Dave Highley had, of course, left UHMBT for Noble's Hospital himself, so I took myself off for a heart-to-heart chat with him.

Sitting in Noble's ICU office with Dave and a welcome coffee, my concerns grew further. Dave had no recollection of the phone call either, and whilst we agreed that neither of us could possibly accurately recall the events of late 2014 from the perspective of six years later, the sequence of events portrayed in these emails made no sense whatsoever to either of us.

And also, how was it possible that these emails had ended up almost instantly in the hands of the GMC? Niche had immediately and categorically denied that anyone in the investigatory team had passed them on. But that meant they could only have been passed on from someone else who had both intimate knowledge of the case and the investigation. Someone outside the immediate investigative team clearly had it in for me and hadn't wasted a second in using these emails to create maximum trouble.

Even more disturbed by these latest developments, I received a call from Professor Alison Birtle that evening. Alison had, of course, been my only NHS witness at the employment tribunal, an act of loyalty and commitment to myself and NHS standards that I hadn't forgotten. Alison's husband – Steve, is an IT expert and she herself is extremely well versed in cyber issues. My voice trembling, I took her through this latest development. *After all,* I told her, *emails don't lie, do they?* There surely couldn't be any possible explanation other than the up-front fact that I'd simply forgotten about Mr Read's desperate position.

Alison was not even remotely impressed with my logic and initial assessment of what had happened.

For heaven's sake Peter.... Sometimes, I'm really bowled over by your work ethic and standards, but at other times I simply cannot believe how utterly naive and gullible you are.... You don't honestly, really believe all that do you?

I had to concede that, well, um...ahhh...yes, I did think of emails as being inviolable.

I was then on the receiving end of a crash course on email tampering, hacking, spoofing, spear phishing, backdating etc. from

127

Alison. Clearly, her impressions of me and my naivety were pretty much bang on the mark, at least in my knowledge of electronic media and digital messaging.

I urgently needed to investigate this a little further but, first of all, I needed to see these emails and their associated headers[7] with my own eyes.

Niche were not prepared to supply copies of the evidence to me. Pointing out that they were the property of the NHS, I was advised that I would now need to apply to the Trust in order to be given a copy. Frustratingly, I was then informed that this would have to go through their Data Protection Act procedures, which would take a good number of days.

Several agonising days later, I did finally get a PDF copy of the two emails and headers. However, I was also keen to know some more of the electronic background to the messages.

UHMBT confirmed that there were currently several copies of these emails in existing accounts, including those of Mr A, Mr B and Mr Cutting.

However, in the process, they also accidentally revealed rather more than they meant to about the digital background.

Two of the six relevant accounts no longer exist....

That didn't have much impact when I first read the UHMBT statement. But when I went back to it, this fact didn't make sense either.

Mr Cutting, Mr B and Mr A are still employed at UHMBT. As is Angela.
Heidi left in about 2017, so her account will have been erased. Therefore, by simple deduction, the other erased account must be...mine!

But how could that possibly be either? As soon as any litigation or judicial process is commenced, or even anticipated, any individual or organisation has an absolute, mandatory and rigorous legal duty

---

[7] The intrinsic electronic data that comes attached to each email.

to preserve <u>all</u> evidence. Since late 2016 and even before I'd left, my old UHMBT email account had been continuously subject to multiple ongoing and overlapping judicial and legal processes and enquiries involving the GMC, CQC and an employment law tribunal. How, and when, could it possibly have been illegally deleted?

UK law could not possibly be clearer on this point.

Under the Civil Procedure Rules of the Courts of England and Wales it is essential for parties contemplating or involved in litigation...to review (and, as necessary amend or suspend) any document retention policies so that no relevant documents are deleted, overwritten or updated (still less permanently destroyed).

It is important to note that the Civil Procedure Rules define 'documents' very broadly...also specifically electronic documents...to include e-mails and other electronic communications...word-processed documents, information on databases, documents that are readily accessible from computer systems, including 'deleted' items, electronically recorded and stored information obtainable from all portable electronic devices and media...information stored on servers and back-up systems and metadata and other embedded data which is not typically visible on screen or a print-out.

Note also that the Courts of England and Wales are able to make very intrusive orders with a view to investigating what a party may have done with relevant documents, should it or the other party suspect that certain documents have been destroyed after litigation was contemplated. Failure to preserve all potentially disclosable documents when litigation is contemplated may also give rise to very serious sanctions, including costs sanctions, the striking out of a party's particulars of claim or defence...and/or the drawing of adverse inferences as to the contents of those documents.

As soon as litigation is contemplated, a prospective party to that litigation must inform all those who might hold any relevant documents under the control of that prospective party of their duty to preserve such documents.[8]

---

[8] www.bristows.com/about-us/compliance-information/duty-to-preserve-documents/.

From: Duffy, Peter
Sent: 13 October 2020 11:24
To: Aaron Cummins

Dear Aaron

I thought that I ought to update you on some of the developments of late last week and over the weekend…. I'll also forward my severe reservations on to the GMC.

Thank you for the email headers and emails which arrived last Wednesday afternoon…what I saw concerned me sufficiently that I approached our IT department. They then referred me on to the Manx Department for cyber-security.

Having analysed the email headers, the Manx cyber-security expert suggested that this was not a matter for them…but instead suggested that I should involve the relevant authorities back in England, which I did yesterday….

My concerns are several. Whilst I'm certainly no IT expert…there is at least one aspect of the headers which troubles me and…needs to be looked into further. I am also troubled by the email contents and the individuals that they were copied to, which do not make sense. Not only are there serious factual errors in both emails, but…the inclusion of these facts clearly raises the suspicion that these emails have been produced considerably more recently than purports to be the case.

Additionally, having taken informal advice over the weekend from several IT experts, no one believes that these emails could have credibly remained entirely undetected by the Trust over a 5½ year period.

I do not accept the explanation that the second email of the 29th only contained 'Mr R' and hence would have been undetectable. Mr Peter Read's full and correct name and accurate unique RTX identifier were both clearly contained within the text of both emails and should have been instantly identifiable, even on the most basic search. The Microsoft search facility reliably and repeatably picks up such details anywhere in an email string and indeed in attached documents. It is utterly inconceivable that...both of these emails, sitting in full-view with Peter's (Mr Read's) correct name and unique identifier, in six different accounts in 11 different forms, marked up as URGENT and high-priority, nevertheless defied search after search including manual, electronic and at least two specific FOI (Freedom of Information) related email searches for nearly 6 years!

Not one of the IT contacts that I have spoken to believes this to be anything other than entirely impossible.

The only credible explanation for the fact that these two emails have suddenly and mysteriously come to light and been passed on (just at the point where both Niche and the GMC are investigating Peter's case), is that they have been introduced at a very much later date.

As per my previous request, I'd be very grateful indeed if I could receive each individual email and header for all of the various recipients; this totalling seven emails in total (allowing for the erasure of my and Heidi's accounts)....

Finally, in my previous correspondence I asked when my account had been erased, who by and for what reason? The Trust's response was to pass on the standard protocol.... This was not the question that was asked, and I would once again ask if I could be supplied with details as to when my account was closed, who closed it and what the reasons behind this were?

Events are moving apace, and I would therefore be extremely grateful, particularly since my requests for information now go back nearly a month, for your urgent attention to the above issues.

Thank you very much in advance.

Yours sincerely
Peter Duffy

The response came three days later.

From: Aaron Cummins
Sent: 16 October 2020 17:53
To: Duffy, Peter
Subject: Emails Request

Dear Peter,

I have spoken to our internal team and they have confirmed that we have adhered to all our Trust policies. We have shared your concerns with NHS England/Improvement for their consideration....

We must be mindful of not conducting further investigations concurrently to that underway for NHS England/Improvement, as this could undermine the effectiveness of the independent review they have commissioned. I am therefore unable to send more information about the emails/email headers.

I am aware that we responded to your question about the reason that your email account was erased in the response to your FOI. This was in line with standard practice/policy. However, I asked our team if we can identify who erased it and when and can advise that it was erased as part of the standard protocol and that this was undertaken by our IT/I3 department. We attempted to identify an exact date, but this has not been possible. We do know that the account was deleted between November 2017 and April 2018. It was not deleted earlier than this due to suspension of deleting whilst the Kirkup Review was underway. The suspension of deleting email accounts was lifted in 2017.

Best wishes
Aaron Cummins

So, my account had seemingly been permanently erased either in the last two months of 2017, or the first few months of 2018.

Employment tribunals are, of course, a court of law, yet this had happened right at the point where all of our employment tribunal enquiries, concerns and preliminary hearings over lack of disclosure and hiding of evidence had been reaching a climax, where multiple searches of my account had been ongoing and where my account was also at the centre of three ongoing GMC reviews as well as ongoing CQC scrutiny. What was even worse, not only had my account seemingly been illegally erased, but UHMBT could only offer a guesstimate to within a few months as to when it had been illegally deleted in defiance of UK law.

What on earth was going on at the time? I mused. *How come UHMBT hadn't protected the account from tampering or followed any of the precautions for the archiving of data used by other large organisations? Surely, with everything that had been going on then, including the legal requirements, implications for the coroner and issues over an avoidable death, the account should have received the digital equivalent of being surrounded by a 24-hour guard, machine guns and barbed wire? Yet somehow, someone had quietly erased a whole decade's worth of evidence – thousands and thousands of potentially pivotal emails without leaving any trace of how or when it had been done....*

This, in my opinion, was no accident. It was the digital equivalent, right in the middle of several judicial processes, enquiries and searches for evidence, of covertly getting several filing cabinets full of potentially vital evidence for a forthcoming legal case and several other enquiries, and then methodically feeding every last bit of it into the shredder.

The text below is taken from the *NHS Corporate Document and Records Management Policy of 2017*, and also the *Records Management Code of Practice for Health and Social Care 2016*.

The emphasis is my own.

<u>NHS Corporate Document and Records Management Policy</u>
18th September 2017

Records involved in Investigations, Inquiries, Litigation and Legal Holds

*5.8.1A Legal hold, also known as a litigation hold, document hold, hold order or preservation order is an instruction directing employees to preserve (and refrain from destroying or modifying) certain records and information (both paper and electronic) that may be relevant to the subject matter of a pending or anticipated lawsuit, investigation or inquiry. <u>**Organisations have a duty to preserve relevant information when a lawsuit, investigation or inquiry is reasonably anticipated**</u>. Staff must immediately notify the assigned Corporate Records Manager if they have been notified of a Litigation, Investigation or Inquiry or have reasonable foresight* *of a future Litigation, Investigation or Inquiry as this could result in records being held beyond their identified retention period.*

Records Management Code of Practice for Health and Social Care 2016.

Email and Record Keeping Implications

One of the most important, yet often neglected, containers of information are the email accounts of staff, which is why it deserves a special mention....

Automatic deletion of email as a business rule may constitute an offence under Section 77 of the FOIA (Freedom of Information Act) *where it is subject to a request for information even if the destruction is by automatic rule.*

The Courts' civil procedure rules 31(B) also require that a legal hold is placed on any information including email when an organisation enters into litigation. Legal holds can take many forms and records cannot be destroyed if there is a known process or an expectation that records will be needed for a future legal process. *This may include national or local inquiries, criminal investigation, and expected cases of litigation or records that may be requested under FOI or subject access. This means that no records can be destroyed by a purely automated process without some form of review whether at aggregated or individual level for continued retention or transfer to a place of deposit.*

In addition to the breaches of the law that had gone on here, there would have been all sorts of searches going on throughout late 2017 and also throughout 2018, with the three employment tribunal hearings and a preliminary hearing heading towards us for just for starters. I'd put in at least two Freedom of Information/Data Protection Act requests in 2016 and 2017, and in late 2017 and early 2018 there had been multiple legal requests from Gateley's for more information to inform the forthcoming employment tribunal. It was totally impossible to believe that, towards the end of this process, no one happened to notice that the email account at the very centre of the case – a case that by summer 2018 was now attracting significant attention in the national media, just happened to have been abruptly and illegally erased. A good number of people in UHMBT <u>must</u> have been aware of this. They could hardly have missed it! Yet, seemingly, everyone had stayed silent, and the judicial process and the Manchester Employment Tribunal panel had proceeded to their final conclusions in late 2018 in complete ignorance of the fact that a major, illegal and industrial sized act of evidential spoliation and destruction had happened, right under their noses and right at the very core of the case. An unlawful act which would potentially have carried massive ramifications, for the tribunal outcome, awarding of potential costs and, most importantly, the verdict itself.

And how utterly outrageous of UHMBT executives to authorise Capsticks Solicitors to threaten costs against myself, whilst quietly concealing the fact that their own organisation had carried out an act of evidential destruction that could and probably should have resulted in the awarding of costs in the opposite direction. (Part III, chapter 3).

Why did no one intervene and try and recover the account at the time? Surely if this had been an accident then strenuous attempts to retrieve it would have been made, as soon as the erasure was discovered and before the account was overwritten, as would inevitably have happened by now?

And had something gone on in my account? Something added to, tampered with or backdated, that was then covered up with the erasure of the entire account?

Now, well over three years on from the account being destroyed, we'd never know….

Chris Thompson, my solicitor from Gateley's had, at the very start of the litigation in 2016, been crystal clear and very forceful indeed about my absolute duty to preserve and present ALL evidence, even if it harmed my case. I'd spent many evenings going back through all my evidence and had been scrupulous in disclosing everything, even where I had suspicions that it might be twisted round and used against me. It was inconceivable that UHMBT wouldn't have been aware of their identical responsibilities and wouldn't have been warned about these obligations by their own legal team from Capsticks.

And how, I mused, *could finding out the truth about the integrity of these emails possibly compromise Niche's enquiries?* Surely, if this enquiry was to be independent and neutral, then it was absolutely vital that only proven and authenticated evidence should be included? The investigation would be massively enhanced, not compromised by getting all the facts out and seeking the absolute truth about these now extremely dodgy looking emails.

If these were forgeries – the digital equivalent of tampering with, or adding to the medical notes, and they ultimately influenced Niche's thinking, made it into the UHMBT urology report and the NHS England investigations into Peter Read's death, and were then wrongly used as being an accurate reflection of what had happened, then the whole process would be corrupted, misled and rendered useless and a complete waste of public money.

And surely, I thought to myself, the whole point of this new examination of the evidence was to fearlessly uncover what had gone on and get to the unfettered, unbiased truth.

Wasn't it?
But then again, all those warnings....
And the anonymous tip-off about evidence being tampered with....
And an alert that at least one person in the Trust wanted to see me in jail...?

———————

THERE WAS ONE PERSON LEFT at UHMBT who I felt I could trust, call and talk to about this evidence – Colin Cutting, who had been copied into both emails. However, at the time I wasn't too bothered by the email of the 26th. It was the one from the 29th that was giving me sleepless nights.

I spoke to Colin after work, sitting in my darkened car in Peel's central car park, waiting with bated breath whilst Colin scrolled back, in real time through his email records. It seemed to take forever to get to December 2014 but was probably no more than a minute or so.

That's odd.... Are you sure of that date? 29th December 2014?
Yeah, that's right Colin.... You were copied in to the second email. 4pm-ish....

I felt like I was going to be sick....

No...no...it's definitely not here. I certainly don't remember any emails like that and it's definitely not in my account for that afternoon. I'm sure I'd have remembered and followed up on any emails like that....
Oh, hang on Peter...there's another email that I received from you earlier that afternoon; that's here, so I was clearly getting emails from you, but definitely nothing about Mr Read.

Relief flushed through me. I realised I'd not been breathing whilst Colin had been scrolling back and forth through the list. Gasping in great, sobbing breaths, it felt like a huge weight had been lifted from me.

You're sure? Definitely? Absolutely certain? You wouldn't have deleted it or something?
Yes, certain, came the answer back. And no. Colin confirmed that he'd never, ever have deleted such an email, nor did he have any recollection of ever seeing such an email. Pointing out that he was clinical lead and head of department at the time, far from deleting such an email, he was clear that he'd meticulously read and retained all clinical emails from this period, and, as departmental head, would have remembered and followed up an *URGENT* and 'high priority' email involving a critically sick ICU patient requiring immediate emergency urological surgery.
How sure can you be that you wouldn't have deleted it? 95%? 99%...?
100% certain, came the answer.
It's not there, and I'd never, ever have deleted something like this.

CHAPTER FIFTEEN

AfPP

IN THE MIDST OF ALL this turmoil and anxiety, it was impossible to feel in control of anything. Blown about helplessly by events like some rudderless sailing ship in a storm, all I could do was to try and stay afloat, cling on to my life and sanity and concentrate on the hear-and-now. Most of all, I was desperate to try and keep my clinical concentration.

Straight after the Niche interview I'd gone immediately to theatre for an emergency case (ironically, an obstructed kidney case) only for the anaesthetist to ask me several times if I was *OK* and fit to operate, so shocked, pale and shaken did I look. Mercifully, family and friends were both sympathetic and supportive, and Peter Read's daughters, Karen and Nicola were also absolutely solidly behind me, despite these new revelations. Somehow, I managed, as far as I'm aware, to stagger through the daily clinical work and sleep deprived nights without any major clinical errors. And, after a few more self-destructive wobbles, I managed to put a reasonably safe distance between myself and further suicidal impulses.

However, right now, on top of all the clinical work and anxieties about the new evidence against me, there was another thing to address.

I'd had much welcome support from the AfPP (Association for Perioperative Practice) and, in response to an editorial from their President Tracey Williams, I'd agreed to do a Saturday morning webinar. Originally billed as an annual conference lecture in York, but cancelled on account of COVID, the on-line presentation was scheduled for a Saturday morning in September.

As conceded in *Whistle in the Wind*, I am probably the world's most nervous and hopeless public speaker and, with the unfamiliar technology of a webinar to cope with, slides to prepare and a necessary theme to try and keep the audience's attention, my anxiety levels ratcheted up another notch. However, I'd undertaken to carry out the on-line lecture and I was determined not to let the AfPP down.

Running through the presentation in my office at Noble's Hospital that Saturday early morning, perhaps half an hour before the webinar was due to start, I was still trying unsuccessfully to relegate the new email evidence to the back of my mind when my mobile went off unexpectedly.

Oh no…. What now…?

Answering and simultaneously thanking my lucky stars that it hadn't gone off during the lecture, it turned out to be the Manx Lieutenant-Governor's office. Would I be free to take a call later that morning?

We agreed a time for after the end of the webinar and I shoved this to the back of my mind too and concentrated on the presentation. *They'll probably be asking me to lecture their staff on male health or something*, I wearily reflected. *Just what I needed….* Switching the phone firmly off, I forgot all about it.

Thankfully the webinar seemed to go well, despite my nerves and distractions. There were some excellent questions, including one particularly penetrating one from Dr James Brown, quoted at the beginning of the book.

Winding down with a chat and debrief with my hosts after the end of the event, I was astonished and flattered to hear that some 600 people had logged in for the event. The AfPP seemed happy with the presentation and I was equally relieved to have got through it without glitches and in blissful ignorance of the number of people registering.[9]

---

[9] The webinar is still available to watch at https://www.youtube.com/watch?v=-dSfLmn2iPc.

Switching on my mobile, I sat and tried to relax, the unbearable emails once more forcing their presence on me. I felt so weary and sleep deprived that even standing up and walking to the car to drive back to Peel seemed like far too much effort.

And then my phone went off again. And now, it wasn't the Isle of Man Lieutenant-Governor's office, it was the Lieutenant-Governor himself....

Caught completely by surprise, I had no idea of what to say, or even how to address the Lieutenant-Governor personally (*Your Excellency* is the answer). I'd never before come remotely close to such a high-ranking official of the Crown. Under the circumstances and caught completely unawares, one syllable grunts and brevity seemed the best defence for my shock and ignorance.

As it happened, brevity wasn't a problem, as the Lieutenant Governor rapidly rendered me speechless anyway.

Are you sitting down and on your own Mr Duffy? Yes? Good. I'm happy to inform you that Her Majesty the Queen has agreed to the award of Member of the Order of the British Empire to you. MBE...for your efforts during the COVID crisis.

Perhaps spurred on by the shocked, disbelieving silence on the other end of the line, he added...

Were you by any chance expecting this?
No? Well, that's good. I always think that those who are completely taken by surprise with these awards are perhaps the most deserving....

I think that we might have exchanged a few more pleasantries before ringing off, but I have no clue what they were. I couldn't have been more shocked if the Lieutenant Governor had climbed out of the phone and thrown a bucket of iced water over me. All I recalled was that I shouldn't speak to anyone about it until the official announcement on October 9th.

Sagging back in the office chair (thank goodness I really had been sitting down) I tried to take stock of the situation. I really didn't feel like I deserved any award, far less an MBE. After all, there were many others on the Isle of Man who'd worked just as hard as me, and thousands of front-line NHS staff across the UK who'd had a far worse time of it. And our own COVID outbreak had lasted only a few months, but across much of the world, the battle to save lives was still very much ongoing.

And I was still struggling to come to terms with my own terrible failings over Peter Read's case.

With a kaleidoscope of whirling, fragmented thoughts, contradictions and clashing emotions spinning round in my head, accompanied by another towering headache, I crept off back to Peel, let myself into the flat, locked the door, climbed into bed fully dressed and firmly pulled the duvet over my head.

It was all just getting far, far too much....

CHAPTER SIXTEEN

More Questions

OF COURSE, EMAILS CAN DISAPPEAR without trace, but, after my telephone call to Colin Cutting, it seemed vanishingly unlikely that a simple internal email in UHMBT's usually highly reliable internal NHS email system would go completely missing, especially when Colin had clearly been receiving other emails from me without problems that afternoon. And I still couldn't get my head around the fact that my account had been illegally erased in the run-in to the employment tribunal.

Phoning up Dave (one of the group of old junior school friends who had been so supportive in the fallout from the 2018 employment tribunal) increased my concerns still further. As in *Whistle in the Wind*, Dave is blunt and forthright. He's a decent, straightforward man and is also a good deal more worldly wise than I am, and just happens to have an extremely good background in IT.

His explanation was instantaneous.

I reckon they've been sent more recently from an external server Pete, and backdated to make them appear that they were sent in 2014. It's that easy, even in an internal intranet system like Morecambe Bay's. Pretty much anything digital or electronic in that kind of system can be tampered with or overwritten, including the headers. Whatever else you do, for heaven's sake don't accept ownership or responsibility for them.

Karen and Nicola – Peter Read's daughters, had clearly been independently thinking through the issue of these new emails and having similar reservations, particularly after my distraught and desperate phone call to them. The family had been in regular and anxious contact with the Royal Lancaster Infirmary's ICU about their father's deteriorating condition on the afternoon of the 29th December 2014, just at the time that the second email was supposedly sent. There had been absolutely no mention whatsoever of a telephone call, theatre, or a review by myself that evening. Furthermore, Nicola had visited her father sometime after work in the early evening. Once again, there had been no mention of any possibility of a review by myself or theatre that evening, or any signs of preparation for theatre. The ICU team had, at the time of Nicola's visit and according to the medical notes, seemed convinced that, as the daytime on-call urology consultant hadn't got back to them with an updated strategy for imaging or emergency surgery that day, the working urological action plan therefore continued to be surgery on my elective (non-emergency) operating list the following day, as per my original handwritten documentation from Friday 26th. Of course, this completely contradicted the information contained in the second of these now extremely dubious looking emails.

Raising even more questions, Karen told me that the family had themselves made a 'Subject Access Request' for all emails relating to their father's case. Made under the stipulations of the Data Protection Act, the request had been made in late 2018 and had been for all emails relating to Peter Read from 28th December 2014 on. The email of the 26th therefore wouldn't have met the criteria, and my account had, of course, been erased by then, so no opportunity to find the outgoing email of the 29th in my own UHMBT emails either.

But searching in the accounts of the other relevant consultants should have thrown up at least three copies of the second email, with the first email attached too. Probably six copies, as UHMBT had searched on both Peter Read's name and his unique RTX hospital number, both of which were present in the attachment to the email of the 29th December.

Karen confirmed that, whilst UHMBT had complied with the Read family's request, had searched and had turned up a good deal of other information, there was no sign of any of the multiple copies of the email of the 29th that would most certainly have been retrieved. Yet there was no logical reason for UHMBT to defy the law, behave dishonestly and decide to withhold the emails. Quite the opposite, in fact. A good number of people would undoubtedly have relished drawing me into the circle of responsibility for Mr Read's death.

———————

AT THIS POINT and after Alison's observations and impromptu tutorial, together with Dave's immediate response, and the fact that searches for the Read family in late 2018 had failed to find any trace of these emails, it seemed appropriate to do some proper due diligence on the black art of email tampering and electronic backdating.

The results truly astonished me. Hacking, data tampering and fake emails were something rare and only ever happened to famous people or huge companies. Wasn't that right? And surely these practices were confined to just a small handful of seedy, disreputable hackers, crouched in some mouldy, dank basement in a far-off lawless country?

The answer was a resounding no. Quite the opposite. As I learned with just a few clicks on my laptop, hacking and electronic fakery is now a worldwide multi-billion dollar industry, with organisations openly advertising on the internet; shiny, polished websites, payment in US dollars via PayPal, results, and both undetectability and discretion guaranteed. It was even possible to have a trial hack to demonstrate the hacker's prowess, and your money held in escrow (an impartial third party account) and only released to the hacker once you are entirely satisfied with the results. Some sites even claimed that it wasn't illegal.

Most staggering of all was how cheap it was. I'd assumed that a 'pro' hack would cost many thousands of dollars, probably tens of thousands if it involved a corporate account. But Dell Computer's contemporary report on worldwide hacking quoted the going rate for a professional private hack at about $140, and $500 for a corporate hack. Furthermore, it seemed that pretty much every form of common electronic storage or transmission was ridiculously vulnerable to hacking, overwriting, backdating or just plain old erasure (as had happened to my old NHS account), including email headers. I also learned that the majority of corporate hacks are 'inside' jobs, carried out, with or without outside assistance, by an employee or manager with a grudge, something to hide or a reason to tamper with evidence.

There were even blogs, describing quite brazenly and in detail how to backdate emails by changing internal computer clocks, so that, for example, a student, told that they had missed a deadline to submit work to a teacher could, with a bit of luck, backdate the work into the teachers account, thereby seeming to hit the deadline and leaving the unsuspecting teacher questioning their own sanity.

...Just like myself....

It was a deeply sobering read, and it seemed to be the appropriate moment to take my by-now overwhelming concerns about the legitimacy of these emails back to Niche.

Substantiating my concerns even further, another conversation with Colin – this time about the email of the 26th, revealed that this particular email did exist in Colin's in-box. However, closer scrutiny revealed yet another anomaly. Whilst the email of the 29th didn't exist in Colin's in-box for the 29th, it was there as an attachment to the email of the 26th. Three days before it was supposed to have been created. Hoping desperately that Colin Cutting's account might hold the key to what had or hadn't gone on in 2014 and since, and with Colin unable to explain the disarray in his inbox in relation to these emails, I passed on my findings to Niche Consulting.

The fallout was for Colin to promptly receive a disciplinary reprimand from UHMBT and instructions to write a reflection in his annual appraisal on his role in assisting me with my questioning the authenticity of these emails. Clearly, some people close to the urology investigation were extremely keen to ensure that these emails and the radically new clinical evidence in them were not discredited, and that I receive no further assistance in querying the legitimacy of this information.

AFTER MY PERSISTENT EXPRESSIONS of concern and in late 2020, Niche instigated an IT assessment of the emails, reporting back to me in a confidential report. They were clearly unhappy with me for querying the authenticity of the emails which, I was now being told, would be used as evidence against me in their *Final Report* to NHS England and to the family of Peter Read. I was further advised that I was making *very serious allegations* by questioning their authenticity, a statement which, in my fear-filled and agitated state sounded sufficiently ominous to very nearly persuade me to drop my expressions of concern altogether and simply admit my responsibility.

Regrettably, I am not allowed to divulge any of the Niche IT report, which was *highly confidential*. However, fervently hoping for a detailed cybercrime investigation to include interrogation of server logs, an on-site review of internal IT security, an explanation for the data breach and erasure of my account in late 2017/early 2018 and a summary of any other evidence of account tampering, as referred to in the anonymous tip-off, I was very disappointed. Furthermore, it seemed that UHMBT had received several weeks warning of the IT review and there was therefore ample time for anyone with something to hide to make sure that the digital evidence trail was squeaky clean.

It was I felt, for these reasons, a flawed and superficial review and an opportunity lost and, even then, Niche's overall conclusion that, on balance, the emails appeared to be probably genuine didn't exactly contain a ringing endorsement of their authenticity.

CONCLUDING MY INCREASING CONCERNS to Niche on 15th November 2020, in the face of their continuing belief in the emails and as part of a much bigger piece of work, I stated:

In summary, I think that we can therefore conclude with extreme confidence that these emails are evidence of nothing more than yet more attempts to force words and actions upon me that I would never countenance, and to once again create confusion and disarray over attempts to establish the true version of events, a tactic that has proved to be only too successful on numerous occasions in the past.

As any kind of reliable evidence, they would undoubtedly be struck out of any judicial process a dozen times over.

Going on, I detailed some 27 reasons to suspect the authenticity of the emails, pointing out that each and every single one of these anomalies would need to have happened for the emails to be authentic.

So, to summarise, in order to believe in the authenticity and legitimacy of these emails, one would have to believe that ALL of the following happened:

1. *I spoke to Peter (Read) after meeting his family about expediting his elective stent change on Friday 26th, and, despite the general surgeons planning for discharge, assessed him as unfit for emergency weekend intervention (something that clearly was not true) in a situation where there was no emergency, and then*

2. *I somehow managed to predict, 12 hours before it became evident, that Peter had a blocked stent and*

3. *Having assured the family that I would try and get Peter on to Monday's or Tuesday's lists and having documented this in the notes, I then went back on this without telling them and only booked Peter for the Tuesday and*

4. *Having detailed a clearly clinically inadequate management plan (bearing in mind the documentation in this email that Peter was deteriorating and had a blocked stent), I then unnecessarily copied a colleague into the email who I knew was actively searching for any clinical errors that I might make and*

5. *Sent two emails to two people in the waiting list office that I would not normally have used. Following this, three days later*

6. *I received an emergency call about Peter from Dr Highley, despite not being on duty, a call neither of us can recollect and which was not documented in the notes and then*

7. *Failed to act on the extreme urgency of this, instead instituting a hopelessly inadequate plan to simply review Peter after the clinic, thus guaranteeing that the Royal College guidelines would be missed, despite the immediate availability of two colleagues in the RLI. We must also accept that I*

8. *Wasted time on an email where, during working hours I would pretty much invariably use the phone and sort things out directly with the waiting list office and*

9. *Then used phrases which I cannot explain or would not normally use, also that I*

10. *Didn't ask for any imaging* (scans) *despite my extreme efforts next morning and that I*

11. *Documented the wrong kind of inotrope* (adrenaline-like drugs). *Then it is necessary to believe that I*

12. *Forgot about Peter altogether, so much so that I went to ward 33 the following morning to see if he had been put on Mr Rowbotham's list. We then have to believe that*

13. *Dr Highley never chased me up or attempted to contact me again, despite my commitment to attend and despite the fact that he was on ICU until 2am that morning.*

14. *The two emails to the waiting list office went entirely unanswered and un-acted upon, despite being marked urgent and, in the latter one, high importance and being sent in working hours. Then...*

15. **Mr A** *and* **Mr B** *decided not to act on the emails, despite their efforts to find evidence of clinical errors on my part and despite the fact that these two emails gifted them not one but two open goals, and then*

16. *One of the two emails mysteriously travelled back in time, being sent on the 29th December 2014, but arriving three days earlier, in Mr Cutting's inbox for the 26th, the date when I sent the original email...*

17. *And the other email that Mr Cutting was sent was equally mysteriously deleted without being read, despite Colin's diligence on checking and filing all departmental emails. After this...*

18. *The extensive literature review for the Royal College of Surgeons enquiry entirely missed the existence of 11 copies of these emails and*

19. *I myself entirely missed both copies in my sent box during my extensive search of incoming and outgoing emails during my last few weeks of employment. We then have to believe that*

20. *The enquiries made for the CQC also missed all 11 copies of these emails, despite them being liberally peppered with triggers and alerts which should have instantly revealed their presence and*

21. *The emails also hid from discovery during my requests for evidence from UHMBT including requests for all correspondence with* Mr A *and* Mr B. *On top of this, we also must believe that*

22. *The Trust's legal team, despite doing some incredibly detailed manual and automated trawls through all my and other people's sent and received emails, entirely missed this very important evidence despite all of the alerts and triggers, scattered through at least nine copies and five internal accounts, and despite both emails being marked up as urgent, with most of them also being marked HIGH IMPORTANCE. And that*

23. *These multiple email copies also managed to hide from discovery during the searches for evidence that were carried out in the legal fallout from 'Whistle in the Wind'. In addition to all of the above, we somehow need to continue to believe that*

24. *The second email managed to continue to hide from discovery again during the email search carried out at the request of Mr Read's family.... We then must believe that*

25. *These emails still continued to hide from discovery during the course of the revised RCA report, and only finally came to light*

26. *As a consequence of a question from yourselves, to which the correct answer would have been a simple 'no' and which didn't ask for any additional information.*

27. *And all this coming after we were explicitly warned in February about internal evidence tampering, and with internal IT governance in UHMBT seeming to be non-existent.*

Sadly, my protestations cut no ice and were rejected out of hand. Clearly, when it came to disallowing these emails as evidence against me, I'd need even harder substantiation, and I'd also need to clear the time and space in my evenings and weekends to do all the investigative legwork and due diligence myself.

––––––––––

CIRCUMSTANTIAL EVIDENCE, like the contradictions between the medical and nursing notes and the emails, the disarray in Colin's otherwise meticulous inbox, the very suspicious alerting of the GMC to their presence and the fact that the family's account contradicted both emails was all very helpful. Indeed, combined with the facts above, it would very likely have been more than enough to get the emails disallowed from any judicial process. However, it now seemed abundantly clear to me that this was no longer an investigation being run on the grounds of fairness, impartiality, judicial standards of rigour and best practice.

I needed <u>proof,</u> not just circumstantial evidence. Ideally, diamond-hard, documented, indisputable verification that these emails hadn't existed in the months and years after 2014, either outgoing in my account, or incoming in the accounts of the recipients and therefore could only have come into existence and been backdated into the relevant consultant's accounts much more recently. Protesting about them, and simply pointing out the fact that multiple searches had *presumably, probably,* or *supposedly* taken place that would have found these emails, but without the hard, factual documentation of such searches clearly wasn't enough.

Thinking it all through, it seemed likely that the emails had been created, sent into the relevant accounts and the time-stamps backdated within the previous six to twelve months. After all, we'd had the anonymous tip-off about evidential tampering in late February 2020, and it was also in the weeks before this that the tense and dubious RCA meeting had happened, accompanied by the executive exclamation of *'this is exactly where I didn't want to find us'*. It was here, too, that for the first time, there had been discussions about who had been on-call that Monday evening and the fact that there had been no handover of Peter Read's case, with it subsequently emerging that the on-call person was me. This was, of course, something that had been worked into the second email. Prior to that 2020 RCA meeting, no one seemed to have checked or remembered anything about that on-call commitment, including myself.

It was also at that meeting that one of my ex-colleagues had, it seemed to me, completely changed his story from that originally provided for the coroner. Now, in a clear contradiction to his original evidence that Peter Read hadn't needed emergency surgery over the weekend in question, he was now insisting that Peter Read <u>had</u> needed surgery after all. However, he'd been too unwell to safely undergo an anaesthetic without intensive care backup, and therefore his emergency surgery had had to wait until the Tuesday. Of course, this new version of events – about Peter being unfit for emergency surgery over the weekend was something that had suddenly appeared in the email of the 26th too.

Mulling this over, I could think of a considerable number of people who might have been motivated to covertly expand on these latest RCA statements, minimise the reputational fallout for the NHS and firmly shift the focus of the investigation away from such overt factual inaccuracies.

Also, Peter Read's family's Data Protection Act request to UHMBT in late 2018 had failed to find the email of the 29th, clearly pushing the date of the email's creation into sometime after the end of 2018.

It also now belatedly occurred to me that in autumn and winter of 2019, my ex-colleague (consultant A) had spent what clearly was many weeks and probably hundreds of hours, exhaustively going back and forth through all his email correspondence with me in order to put together the voluminous evidence that he'd forwarded to the GMC (Part I, chapter 5).

He'd obviously been both highly focused and motivated and had picked up a huge array of emails from all the way back to about 2010 including much that was utter trivia and had forwarded many dozens of emails from me and about me to the GMC over a period of several months. Under no circumstance that I could think of could he possibly have completely missed both of these emails in his account from 2014, especially with both clearly sent to him from my own named account, both containing Peter Read's details, both marked up as URGENT, and the second supposedly red-flagged and *high priority* too.

So, these emails <u>must</u> have been backdated into my ex-colleague's accounts sometime after the end of 2019, and probably more recently than that.

Exactly the point where I'd had the tip-off about evidential tampering and a vendetta against myself.

By a process of deduction, to try and prove (as opposed to raising the strong suspicion of) the illegitimacy of these emails, I'd somehow have to come up with a way of formally assessing the contents of either my account, Mr A's, Mr B's or Mr Cutting's account or, in a perfect world, all four of them, as they would have been prior to late 2019.

If these emails were authentic, they would, by necessity, have had to have existed continuously in my account and in the accounts of Mr A, Mr B and Mr Cutting from late 2014, all the way through to the present. If I could somehow prove that they had not – that a documented, rigorous, meticulous search of one or more of these accounts, prior to early 2020, had failed to find these emails despite using the exact and perfect criteria to discover them, then this would be the hard proof and confirmation of backdating and fakery that I needed.

Impossible....

For starters, my own account had been permanently destroyed, would by now be completely overwritten, and UHMBT wouldn't be allowing me within a million miles of it even if it still existed. The same applied to Mr A's and Mr B's accounts. And, of course, Colin had, in no uncertain terms, been warned off giving me any further assistance with my rapidly consolidating suspicions.

I wasn't going to get any third party help either. The UK cyber-crime police had handed the case to the local Lancashire constabulary. However, not unreasonably, and having pointed out the fact that these emails related to events over five years ago, the police clearly felt that impounding servers and carrying out a detailed and forensic IT survey would not be worth the cost to them and disruption to the NHS.

So, I was on my own, thoroughly boxed in and at a dead-end with proof.

But still, I couldn't leave the thought-trail alone. It was as though my subconscious was prodding me and shaking its head in frustration at my obtuseness. Perhaps the truth was right in front of me, and yet I was too distracted with the details to see it.... Or perhaps another part of my subconscious didn't want to have to go back and revisit earlier unpleasantries…?

It was sometime over Christmas 2020 (at about the time that my first musings over a second book were crystallising), that thoughts about proof and evidence, and going back and revisiting the employment tribunal correspondence began to make themselves known. There never was an epiphany or eureka moment. Perhaps, at my age and in the case of the latter, it was just as well.

Instead, just a vague notion, sneaking around at the back of my mind that it might just be worth revisiting this period. I'd (probably deliberately) blocked these thoughts and memories from my waking hours, but I vaguely recalled bad tempered and deeply upsetting exchanges about disclosure of evidence between myself and Gateley's on the one hand, and Capsticks Solicitors and the UHMBT legal team on the other. Perhaps those disclosure requests might throw something up? And all the grumpy exchanges about legal obligations, evidence and disclosure had gone on long after these emails claimed to have been sent, but also well before there were any tip-offs or suspicions of evidential backdating or tampering.

Perhaps this period of legal arguments might be worth closer scrutiny?

I was very well aware that extensive searches for evidence had been done on both sides of the legal argument in 2016 to 2018 and there'd been no sign of these emails then. But UHMBT would, of course, claim that the searches simply hadn't used the correct methods, software or search criteria to find these particular emails, or perhaps there had been *human error*. And, of course, my assurances about the emails being absent from my own account during my personal searches when I left the Trust would carry no weight at all, with Niche or with the NHS. However, there was just a chance that the legal sparring of 2016 to 2018 might reveal more than I could immediately recall.

Resolving to dig out all the old legal emails, one quick search of my email account was enough to put me off, almost forever. The exchanges that I brought up immediately resurrected all sorts of awful memories and I hastily closed them down again. The nights were more than disturbed enough without re-awakening all sorts of awful flashbacks and sickening recollections and, for the moment at least, it seemed sensible to concentrate on trying to enjoy the festive season and precious time with my family and to defer revisiting such toxicity and nastiness until I was back on the island.

By mid-January 2021 though, I'd run out of excuses to put off my search.

Beginning with summer of 2016, I methodically began to work my way forwards through the email exchanges between myself, UHMBT, Capsticks and Gateley's.

And pretty much straight away, I hit paydirt. Not only did I find my original Subject Access Requests for all email correspondence to, from or about myself, *but critically I'd completely forgotten that UHMBT had divulged exactly how they would carry the request out*. Lacking the software to carry out a search through the whole Trust IT system, Information Governance told me that they would search in the individual Microsoft Outlook accounts of, amongst others, Mr A and Mr B *for emails that reference Peter Duffy*.

Bingo....

From: ▇ ▇ (UHMB)
Sent: 14 September 2016 16:00
To: Duffy Peter (UHMB)
Subject: RE: FOI Request

Dear Peter,

I have passed your request onto our Information Governance Manager. They have now confirmed that they now have enough information to proceed with your request.

*Information Governance have asked me to make you aware that they will search the email accounts of the names that you provided (…*consultant A, consultant B…*) for emails that reference 'Peter Duffy' for the time period 01-01-2010 to 14-09-2016 but if any further names are requested following this initial request these will be treated as separate search.*

Once this process is completed, they will let me know and I will contact you to arrange the best way to provide this documentation to you.

If you have any queries regarding the above information, please do not hesitate to contact me.

Kind Regards, ▇

Of course, this meant that any and all emails that had been sent or copied from me to Mr A and Mr B between 2010 and 2016 would register in the searches of their accounts. Testing this out on my own Noble's Hospital Outlook account, I was quickly able to confirm that searching on an individual's name in an Outlook account reliably and consistently brought up all incoming emails from that individual, as well as third party emails in which they were named. So, therefore, if these emails had existed in late 2016/early 2017, UHMBT's response to my Subject Access Request would have brought up the first email from the 26th, recovered from Mr A's account, as well as two copies of the second email of the 29th with the first email attached, as this was supposedly sent to both Mr A and Mr B.

Two problems. Firstly, UHMBT had taken many months to reply to my original request, and, secondly, when I did finally locate their response to the Subject Access Request, they had redacted every single one of the emails found in these accounts to the point where it made a complete mockery of the laws on disclosure (see *Whistle in the Wind,* pages 181-186).

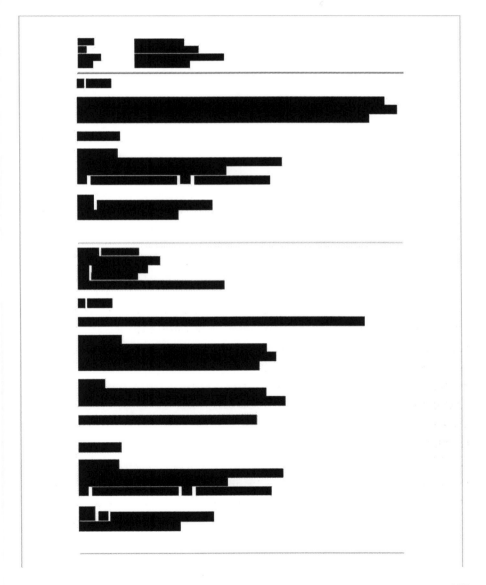

Back to the drawing board.

But wait a minute.... Although UHMBT had indeed erased huge sections, often the entire email string, critically, it was still possible, even in the email evidence that had been completely destroyed, to work out roughly how many people the email had been sent to, how many had been cc'd in, whether the email had a title and whether it had been replied to. Combining this with the layout and spacings of sentences and paragraphs and comparing carefully with the copies of these two very questionable emails that I now had, I could still figure out if these emails really had been received into the accounts of my two ex-colleagues in late 2016 and 2017, even if the emails had been redacted to the point of complete unreadability.

Laboriously working through each of many, many emails, I spent a good number of evenings painstakingly comparing each redacted email provided by UHMBT with the two emails disclosed to Niche and the GMC.

Finally, very late one evening and with a towering headache, I sat back and closed the laptop with a snap and a sigh of relief.

None of the hundreds of redacted emails, featuring my name and electronically extracted from the accounts of Mr A, Mr B and others had the same layout of direct recipients and copied-in recipients as either of the two emails in question, and the layout of the headings and text of the two fakes came nowhere near matching any of the redacted emails that I'd just worked through.

It seemed clear that, in late 2016, UHMBT's detailed, digital searches through Mr A's and Mr B's accounts for emails from me or featuring me had failed to show up any trace whatsoever of the three email copies that would most certainly have been uncovered in such a search.

This at last was good, hard verification of my suspicions; much, much better than the rather softer circumstantial evidence that I'd produced to this point.

I slept a little more soundly that night.

But still the nagging doubts came. I'd already produced a good thirty or so reasons to doubt the validity of these emails. We now knew that there had been an illegal data breach and erasure of my account in late 2017 to early 2018 and, of course, we'd had the very authentic sounding tip-off about tampering with evidence from late February of 2020.

On top of all this, the email from the 29th was missing from Colin's in-box on that day and was also missing from the family's request for emails. And now, we had hard evidence, indeed proof, that a search of Mr A's and Mr B's accounts in late 2016 and early 2017 had failed to show up any trace of these emails that, it was claimed, had been copied to them, were now present in their accounts and which claimed to have been there continuously all the way back to 2014.

Surely, this was now sufficient proof to have these emails rejected as evidence of anything other than evidential spoliation, backdating and indirect tampering with the clinical records?

However, I still had a dread sense that, whatever the Terms of Reference of the urology enquiry had said about evidential rigour, we'd already strayed very far indeed from the kind of robust, strictly impartial and evidence-driven process that had been promised, and deep, in my opinion, into the territory of anti-whistleblower prejudice.

Of course, I was unaware at this point of the full extent of Niche's investigations and can only convey my instincts at the time, but there had been no more interviews with Niche after the two that had nearly sent me under the builder's truck and, from my own perspective, this no longer felt like a rigorous, impartial pursuit of the truth, and rapidly seemed to have degenerated into something with the rigour and impartiality of an old-fashioned feudal witch-hunt.

Niche, NHS England and UHMBT were, I believed, sufficiently wedded to the new and damning implications in these emails that they'd reject my latest findings, based, as they were, on redacted and thus unreadable emails.

I'd better keep searching....

And then, after several more evenings of sifting through old messages and arguments, and re-living old traumas and frustrations – pure, joyful, unadulterated gold....

CHAPTER SEVENTEEN

Proof

I'D FOLLOWED UP MY UNSATISFACTORY late 2016 Subject Access Request to UHMBT in mid-summer of 2017. The employment tribunal was approaching, and it seemed clear that UHMBT would have to do rather better than presenting a UK court of law with a mass of black lines by way of their mandatory evidence disclosure obligations.

On the 30th July 2017, I'd emailed Chris at Gateley's asking him to pass on to Capsticks and UHMBT a further pre-tribunal request for *all communications, emails, recordings, minutes in which I am referenced as Peter Duffy, PD or P Duffy, mentioning or related to myself, from or to or copied to the following individuals....* Within that list of individual accounts were, amongst others, those of Mr A and Mr B.

The request was to supply all documents from July 2017 back to January 2010. This request was supplemented in early February 2018, as the employment tribunal drew ever closer, for *all file notes, informal notes, emails, drafts, letters, meeting notes etc relevant to the issues.* Once again, a list of key individuals, including Mr A and Mr B was provided.

I now recalled that Capsticks and UHMBT had responded to the multiple requests by sending through a huge registered mail packet of paper print-offs, two Lever-arch files worth which subsequently formed the backbone of the 3,500-page *legal bundle* upon which the tribunal evidence, my own witness statement and, subsequently, *Whistle in the Wind* was based. This arrived in late 2017.

Casting my mind back, I'd spent a good many hours sitting in my rented flat in Peel, carefully sorting out this huge mass of paper emails and letters into piles of the very important, relevant and irrelevant. Critically, these two emails of 2014, claiming to have been sent to several of the key individuals should have been recovered many times over in all these multiple searches. Yet, crucially, despite the huge packet of paperwork having supposedly been the sum total of all emails matching the descriptions and specifications provided by me in 2017... *they had been entirely absent from this package too....*

But what came next was much, much better still.

Chris (my solicitor) and I, quite rightly as it turned out, had both had very severe reservations about whether UHMBT were actually obeying civil law and dutifully disclosing all the evidence that was relevant to my case, and that they had available in the accounts of my ex-colleagues. In the end, and out of sheer frustration, we'd requested a preliminary hearing at the Manchester Employment Tribunal to try and force full disclosure from the Trust, as should have already happened under the mandatory legal rules of disclosure.

In response to this and on 19th February 2018, UHMBT, via Capsticks Solicitors, supplied a formal *Skeleton Statement* (a kind of legal statement of truth) to the judge and to the tribunal in respect of the disclosure of evidence.

...I so very very nearly missed it...!

I'd never been required to attend this preliminary hearing – had completely forgotten about it and, late at night, I was tired, disorientated, gritty eyed and sleep deprived. And the attachment in question was just another inconspicuous add-on to just another unexciting looking email.

But, buried in amongst UHMBT's belligerent denials of any withholding of relevant evidence was a formal, legal statement from UHMBT to Judge Batten, the judicial chair of the preliminary hearing.

Capsticks, on behalf of the Trust and in their legal affidavit, listed all the accounts that had been digitally searched by UHMBT for mutual correspondence. My account was there, as was consultant A's, consultant B's and, very importantly, Mr Colin Cutting's too. I'd never asked for Colin's account to be searched, but clearly, the Trust hadn't restricted itself to just searching the accounts that I'd requested back in 2017. There was at least one name there that I didn't recognise at all, and several others in addition to Colin's that I hadn't asked for.

Here, at long, long last, was hard, authenticated proof that the email Outlook accounts of myself, Mr A, Mr B and Mr Cutting had indeed been properly and appropriately searched and electronically interrogated for all mutual correspondence. Furthermore, some 3,000 emails of such mutual correspondence <u>had</u> been discovered, forwarded on and incorporated into the *legal bundle* of evidence, so clearly the searches had been done, and done very rigorously indeed. And these two emails *were not there anywhere, in any of these accounts or searches....*

Better still, Capsticks and UHMBT went on to certify that the possibility of any relevant documentation exchanged between these various accounts between 2010 and 2017 having escaped from being found and disclosed during this process was, in their words *untenable.*

The Respondent (UHMBT) respectfully submits that it has already made a reasonable search of its systems including reviewing the circa 3,000 emails which were referred to by the Claimant in his application which referred to 'Peter Duffy', 'P Duffy' or 'PD' to determine the relevance of those documents....

The Claimant's optimistic belief that there must be more is untenable.

The Respondent has already disclosed correspondence between:

a. *the Claimant;*
b. ████ *;*
c. ██ ██ *; (consultant A)*
d. ████ *;*
e. ████ *;*
f. ████ *;*
g. *Colin Cutting;*
h. ████ *;*

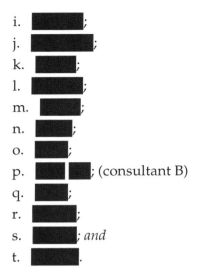

i. ▮▮▮▮;
j. ▮▮▮▮;
k. ▮▮▮;
l. ▮▮▮;
m. ▮▮▮;
n. ▮▮▮;
o. ▮▮▮;
p. ▮▮▮ ▮▮; (consultant B)
q. ▮▮▮;
r. ▮▮▮;
s. ▮▮▮; *and*
t. ▮▮▮.

The documentation disclosed is the extent of documentation that has been located by the Respondent following its search.

Perfect....
Just perfect....

———————

WELL...AT LONG, LONG LAST.

There it is.

Rigorous and, crucially, legally certified and signed off UHMBT IT searches had been done in 2017 to 2018 that had included all emails out of my account, and also, all incoming emails from myself in the accounts of Mr A, Mr B and Mr Cutting from 2010 onwards. Searching in my account would, if these emails were genuine, have revealed five outgoing copies. Two emails to Mr Cutting, two to Mr A and one to Mr B. Searching on Peter Duffy in these latter accounts of the three consultant recipients would have brought up all five incoming copies of the now indisputably fake emails. Searching in

Mr A's, Mr Cutting's and Mr B's accounts for 'P Duffy' would also have brought up yet another five incoming copies.

So, in stark contrast to both the Trust's and Niche's assurances that there had only been one missed opportunity, there had, in fact, been a minimum of fifteen cast-iron, unmissable occasions when over a dozen copies of these fake emails would have been found if they were genuine, just in this one search alone and, once again, *they were completely absent – over and over and over again.*

Whilst I'd been tipped off in 2018 about concerns that UHMBT was hiding important evidence from the tribunal, there was no way that they'd have kept quiet about these emails. After all, between them the two emails offered previously unheard of fig leaves for both Mr A and Mr B, at a time when the Trust was desperately trying to defend them and their actions. Neatly passing a fair bit of the responsibility back to me, it was clear that if UHMBT had found even one solitary copy of these emails in 2017 or 2018, it would have been trumpeted as the lead item in their legal case. Instead, there had never been a whisper, until after the embarrassment and the inconsistent and shifting evidence of the second RCA in early 2020, and the subsequent anonymous tip-off about tampering with evidence.

Here was clear, unequivocal, legally authenticated and certified proof, offered to Judge Batten in a judicial process and in the form of a sworn statement, that what clearly were highly rigorous searches of all of these accounts in late 2017/early 2018, utilising exactly the right search criteria had found not one single copy matching these two forgeries in any of the four relevant accounts.

––––––––––

I SO VERY NEARLY STOPPED at this point.

After all, why on earth go on? What possible further proof could I need? It surely couldn't get any better than this…. A legal, sworn statement after a thorough search, declaring that these emails definitively hadn't existed in any of the relevant accounts in 2018, and made to a judge too?

Thankfully, I decided to keep going a little further, and, if it were possible, even harder proof was still to follow.

Judge Batten, summarising her findings in the preliminary hearing, and amongst other things, formally ordered:

All internal UHMBT documents in respect of the avoidable death issue to be disclosed as is any correspondence with the coroner's office in respect of this matter.

This, of course, legally required the Trust to go back and search all over again in all the relevant accounts for anything relating to Peter Read, the *avoidable death issue* at the centre of the employment tribunal case.

Knowing already from UHMBT's Information Governance email of how the system worked, it was clear exactly what would have happened next. The accounts of all the key individuals would have been searched again on the specifics of Peter Read's name, and then again on his unique UHMBT 'RTX' hospital reference number.

Both of these identifiers were correctly reproduced in these fake emails and, if they had been authentic, I calculated that another 14 copies of these emails would have been found.

Frantically scrolling forward through my email records, I quickly found UHMBT's response to Judge Batten's judicial order. Marked as *PR Pack,* the Trust had duly carried out the searches and had disclosed another roughly 300 pages of further documentation, all of which was subsequently added to the legal bundle.

And the fake emails?

Once again. They were nowhere to be seen….
…absolutely <u>perfect</u> triangulation.

Sitting back and pushing my laptop away, I savoured perhaps 15 minutes of pure silence and absolute peace.

Is this what it's like I thought, *being in the eye of the hurricane?*

It was late; way after midnight, pitch dark outside and very, very cold. The central heating had switched itself off long ago, and the flat had cooled off to the point where my breath hung in the air. The onshore and scalpel sharp winter wind whispered and moaned around the roof and chimneypots; the slates rattled and suddenly I was aware of the distant waves, crunching down onto the sands of Peel beach after their long journey from Ireland. Sitting alone, bitterly cold, and in a little puddle of laptop light, I'd been so engrossed in this new information that the dropping temperature had gone completely unnoticed.

However, I wasn't inclined to do anything other than relish the moment.

Here at last, by a truly extraordinary stroke of luck, and in complete contradiction to the explanations offered by the NHS and Niche, was the absolute hard proof that was needed, and many, many times over too.

For a good number of weeks, I'd been absolutely confident that these emails were fake. But now, we'd gone way beyond confident.

Here was absolute proof.

Clearly, dozens of highly detailed automated trawls had been done through all the relevant individual UHMBT accounts again and again and again between 2016 and 2018. The exact and perfect search criteria to find these emails over and over again had clearly been used, documented and the results formally presented to a legal, judicial process (the Trust had found, by their own admission over 3,000 emails). My own, conservative estimate was that there had been well in excess of 30 rigorous, software driven occasions when the perfect search criteria had definitely been used; when these two emails just couldn't possibly have been missed, and which would have turned up dozens of copies of these two messages, had they existed before the end of 2018.

And no trace had ever been found.

As several IT experts have pointed out to me, computers don't make human-level mistakes, least of all when they're searching for a simple sequence of numbers or letters in a limited dataset, like searching for someone's name or number in an email account. They don't get bored or fed up, bunk off home early, have Friday afternoon episodes or wake up with a hangover. And it was utterly inconceivable that numerous, rigorous digital searches, carried out over many different months, probably by different individuals sitting at different computer consoles through different accounts would have sequentially missed each and every single one of dozens of different opportunities to find these critical emails, whilst accurately finding thousands of others. Emails don't casually slip down the back of the filing cabinet, only to be 'accidentally' rediscovered years later....

They exist – continuously.

Or, as in this case, they don't.

It was exactly, I thought to myself, as though dozens of people had searched diligently and repeatedly through Peter Read's written, paper medical notes for evidence over a period of four years or so. And then suddenly and completely unexpectedly, years on, two new, never-ever-seen-before pages had inexplicably appeared between the existing notes, both entirely changing the narrative and contradicting the other notes.

And all this coming just a few weeks after we'd been tipped off about attempts to interfere with evidence, warnings about a vendetta and a senior manager in UHMBT wanting to see me jailed, and with UHMBT having concealed, for at least two years, the fact that an illegal erasure of my personal email account had taken place prior to the employment tribunal.

Here at last, it was possible to turn the clock back several years; to a time before any tampering, erasures or warnings about evidential spoliation and see exactly what these detailed searches had brought up.

There was no possible or credible explanation other than electronic tampering, backdating and falsification.

These emails had been fabricated and backdated into the record sometime <u>after</u> the Read family's Subject Access search of late 2018 and Mr A's 2019 searches for evidence against me.

I was in the clear....
Thank God...thank God...thank God....

AND THEN, MY HEADY RELIEF and my elated mood, with the release of so many months of terrible pent-up anxiety and stress, began to change and darken. With the foul, acid taste of vomit in my mouth, I began to shiver more and more violently and uncontrollably.

How was it possible that I'd come within a hairs breadth and a split second of ending my own life over these emails – emails purporting to contain hard evidence of clinical errors by myself that I had been repeatedly assured appeared to be genuine, only to find months later, solid, definitive proof that they'd clearly, deliberately and cynically been falsified and backdated into the NHS IT record, seemingly to add *new* clinical information, and mislead, brain wash and gaslight me into believing in my own responsibility for Peter Read's death?

Someone or, almost certainly, a small group of people had, it seemed to me, been very, very devious indeed.

In the run-up to the Niche enquiry, I'd been so suspicious that tampering with the medical notes might happen that I'd even, with the family's permission, photographed them all out. At least one other person that I knew of had been apprehensive enough that, entirely unknown to me at the time, they'd done exactly the same. So there was no way that surreptitiously tampering with the hand-written medical records would have fooled anyone.

But altering the parallel electronic NHS IT evidence?

How clever was that?

For a good number of weeks, I'd been completely duped.

On the other hand, how could it possibly be that the defining and damning evidence to entirely discredit these emails had been there all the time in UHMBT, in plain sight – easily accessible to both the Trust's senior managers and Niche? There must be dozens of emails to and from individuals in UHMBT's HR, IT, governance and legal departments, containing huge amounts of detail of all these different searches, findings and the thousands of emails, and all of them easily accessible. And, of course, the public documents exchanged between UHMBT, Capsticks Solicitors, the judge and the different individuals involved in my employment tribunal hearings.

UHMBT <u>knew</u> that I was a very real suicide risk after the emails had been sprung on me. They'd even tipped off the Manx Medical Director about the clear risk in what, even at the time, had seemed to be a rather cynical bit of virtue-signalling and buck-passing. Yet all the time that they'd been virtuously expressing concern about me taking my own life, they'd also been quietly sitting on hard, legally certified evidence of dozens of searches that would have blown these emails sky-high.

And, of course, instantly removed any risks of self-harm.

Instead, I thought, *I'd been left in a trap with only one obvious way out....*

And I'd come so very close to taking it....

As well as all of this, I'd openly compared Peter Read's death with a case from a few years earlier where a consultant urological surgeon *had* been jailed for a very similar lapse of standards. And here was faked-up evidence that would have placed me squarely in the firing line for a similar outcome.

A possible jail sentence for negligence and medical manslaughter....

And I'd actually admitted my culpability to Niche at my first interview – openly acknowledged my shock at my own neglect, purely on the assurance that these emails appeared genuine. I'd come so terrifyingly close to unconditionally believing in their authenticity, resigning my registration as a consequence and, of course, thereby implicitly acknowledging my guilt and my part in the responsibility for Peter Read's death.

So, if I'd survived the overwhelming and predictable temptation to escape this digital trap in what at the time seemed the only way out possible – ending my own life in disgrace, exactly as UHMBT had foreseen; then, as a fallback, these emails, and my shocked response and confession would have offered the police and the Crown Prosecution Service an open goal. An open and shut case of medical manslaughter based on my own concession of guilt....

Shocked and trembling with horror, I disbelievingly reflected back over the events of the previous sickening and hellish 12 months. It felt just as though I'd been carefully set up.

Manipulated, gaslighted and indeed, carefully and meticulously groomed for some kind of utterly catastrophic outcome.

Dear God...I'd come so unbelievably close to being totally and utterly stitched up....

———————

THINKING BACK, THESE FAKE EMAILS HAD, I was told, caused significant waves within the Trust when they had suddenly, inexplicably exploded into view in late summer 2020. How come not one single person had stepped forward to express their concerns or to point out the overwhelming and conclusive evidence that these emails didn't, at any point, exist throughout the multiple searches, evidence gathering and judicial declarations of 2016 to 2019?

And the GMC had independently come into possession of these emails at almost exactly the same time as Niche. Yet Niche had been immediately crystal clear with me that these emails had not been passed on as a consequence of their own investigation. After more than five years of dozens of negative searches, if these emails were genuine, what was the likelihood of both of these emails being simultaneously and independently rediscovered by chance by two entirely different individuals within days of each other? Especially after the anonymous tip-off, shouldn't this have triggered immediate questions and have instantly invalidated these emails as evidence of anything other than covert evidential tampering?[10]

———————

[10] Shortly before publication of *Smoke and Mirrors*, the GMC confirmed that the emails had not come to them via Niche or UHMBT. Instead, they had, entirely independently it would seem, come into the possession of *another doctor*. They were then forwarded by this individual to consultant B and were then forwarded again to the GMC from consultant B via his medical defence organisation, this happening sometime in August or September 2020, at the same time that UHMBT passed the emails to Niche.

Who from the Trust seemed to have assured both Niche and Peter Read's grieving family that there had only been one missed opportunity to find these emails (that opportunity being the family's Subject Access Request from late 2018), when, in fact that there had been quite literally dozens of opportunities prior to this? And, of course, UHMBT's sworn certification of their non-existence in 2018 to an employment law judge.

Why hadn't Niche done what seemed to me to be the basic, investigative work and asked the obvious questions about the mandatory legal searches to fulfil the NHS's obligations in the run up to the employment tribunal? And why had it fallen to me to go back through UHMBT's own tribunal submissions and do the fundamental, obligatory, due-diligence investigatory background work-up?

And, of course, I'd been warned off – and so very, very nearly put off questioning and researching the authenticity of these emails; told that I was making *very serious allegations* and potentially *compromising the NHS England enquiry.*

How unbelievably cynical that now looked!

How did this fit with an impartial, rigorous investigation? And how could a hugely expensive, taxpayer-funded, supposedly bias-free and independent investigative process, led and overseen by NHS England themselves, have been so corrupted and distorted; incorporating false, backdated, completely misleading and easily disproven evidence against the whistleblower, right from the very start of the process?

And was there anything else that might more recently have been *discovered* and quietly incorporated into the evidence against me? I barely dared to think about the possibilities….

And how was it that, after two interviews which were almost exclusively devoted to these emails, Niche had not taken their enquiries with me any further? There were so many other issues that needed to be investigated, including some which I'd sanitised or glossed over in *Whistle in the Wind* for fear of retaliatory litigation. How could a wide ranging and supposedly independent enquiry have focussed solely on force-feeding these now-discredited emails to me, and go on to ignore all the other evidence that I had to give?

I recalled UHMBT's earnest sounding assurances and the executive promises about *Freedom to Speak Up*, refreshed in the wake of the Kirkup report into the midwifery scandal, that *no whistleblower will lose their job or suffer any detriment....* The exact-same NHS promises that had, of course, been quietly airbrushed out of the Trust's website in the run-up to the tribunal hearings. And now, not only had I lost my job, vocation, family, health, social life and also a six-figure sum despite the tribunal pay-out, but I'd been gaslighted, groomed and brainwashed into coming within a whisker of killing myself, or, failing this, being tricked into admitting my part in the responsibility for Peter Read's death. A responsibility that could easily have led to a striking off, disgrace and a possible prison sentence. And all purely as a result of clearly fake emails, originating from the very same organisation that had made such unequivocal and ultimately, utterly false and misleading promises.

Struggling to comprehend the extremes of enmity and hatred that might have led to this, it seemed that a very deliberate, skilful and well-orchestrated disinformation exercise had taken place.

And I'd come <u>so</u> close, so very, very close to accepting this back-dated version of events as the truth and admitting what seemed to be my clear legal culpability. And so terrifyingly close to completely missing the legal email attachment and official legal affidavit containing this indisputable proof.

And if I had been indoctrinated and gaslighted into killing myself as a consequence of believing these now-entirely discredited and counterfeit emails; psychologically manipulated and groomed into believing in my guilt, the life crushed out of me underneath a speeding truck; snuffed out by a trap primed with false NHS evidence, spin and fabrications, leaving a grieving family, widow, young men, barely out of their teenage years, but now fatherless....

What would have happened next...?

Would senior UHMBT executives and NHS England have contritely come forward, putting out an honest, comprehensive statement to admit that all the time, this huge, monopolistic and manipulative state organisation had possessed hard, defining and triangulated proof that these awful emails were actually counterfeit? Would the NHS have apologised, published the hard proof of fakery contained within their own internal messages, legal files and depositions, exonerated me and generously offered to compensate and indefinitely support the family, bearing in mind the board's original promises, now that the husband and father had killed himself as a direct, predictable and immediate consequence of the UK state health service's own spin, dishonesty, evidential tampering and gaslighting?

Like hell it would have...!

Any remaining internal NHS evidence that disproved these emails, would, I surmised, with a few anonymous clicks of a mouse have been fired into electronic oblivion in the same way as my original email account. My brutally bereaved family would have been pitilessly left to fend for themselves, with only some freshly dug turf and a headstone to remind them of their dead and mutilated ex-surgeon, whistleblower, husband and father. The facts presented in *Whistle in the Wind* would be discredited and the book probably disgraced. Amazon would be robustly approached to withdraw publication, and all the wider issues over candour, safeguarding and speaking up would be simply closed down and killed off.

And an ice-cold, crystal-clear message would have been sent to any other NHS employees considering whether to speak-up.

In the meantime, I could just imagine the slippery and carefully crafted statements that would have been put out.

We deeply regret...sadly...clear, unequivocal evidence implicating him in the clinical negligence issues that emerged over the avoidable death of Patient A...respect the privacy of the family in this moment of loss...integrity of the investigation was of paramount importance...clearly and sadly was unable to reconcile himself with his own share of the failures, neglect and responsibilities in this tragic case....

Of course, my death in late 2020 would have been followed by an inquest.

The balance of his mind was materially affected...the deceased intended his own death; tragic end...unable to face his own responsibility...couldn't resolve being presented with the truth of his own culpability and the possibility of a custodial sentence....

...he did act with that intention which caused his death....

Verdict:

Suicide.

I'm sitting on a hard, uncomfortable wooden chair, at my regular desk in classroom 2M. Casual graffiti and fading ink blots from previous generations of schoolboys define the desk's grainy, work-worn surface.

1975.

The warm afternoon sun is slanting in through the grimy windows, picking out little motes of dust lazily spiralling in the air. A fly is buzzing somewhere. I'm hot and sweaty in my regulation dark woollen school trousers, white shirt and college tie. Everything else seems to be grubby shades of gloss cream, beige or brown. My hair, in teenage defiance of school regulations, reaches well below my collar, Queen's Bohemian Rhapsody is number one in the charts, the newly released Austin Princess is the height of automotive sophistication and the newspapers are full of arguments about football hooligans, IRA terrorists and someone I've never heard of before – Margaret Thatcher, the newly-appointed, first female leader of the conservative party.

She'll never make a mark, we'd all wisely opined during the lunchbreak. Too shrill and self-opinionated. Probably be here today, gone-and-forgotten tomorrow....

But I'm not thinking about any of these things anymore and, despite the heat, stuffiness and testosterone-charged humidity of a class of 30 gangly adolescent boys, all packed together, I'm not sleepy, bored or distracted, like I'd usually be.

Well-thumbed by several generations of acne faced teenagers, I'm entranced by our English literature lesson book. Transported to another world and a very different country.

I'm entirely oblivious to my surroundings.

A truly corrupt, dystopian and frightening future. A totalitarian, monopolistic, unelected state organisation; electronic manipulation and fakery; tampering with and backdating of facts. A snooping, omnipresent, controlling and distrusting national entity. Doublethink – where the organisation can pursue two totally contradictory policies; both, and all at once repudiating morality whilst laying claim to it. A Ministry of Truth which pumps out and backdates organisationally authorised lies to cover up or amend errors of judgement or reputationally uncomfortable facts. A Ministry of Love that oversees the brainwashing, torture and degradation of non-subservient and non-compliant citizens.

Double standards, hypocrisy, spin, treachery and lies, and, at the centre of it all, a very human character, trying to make sense of all the contradictions, never knowing who he can trust and who might, at any moment, betray him. And, of course, ultimately forced, manipulated and indoctrinat-

ed into submission to a despotic entity that behaves, not just as though it owns its subjects, but as though it has an automatic right of possession and make-or-break dominance over them. Controlling, corrupt, narcissistic and ever-watchful, manipulative of thoughts, consciousness and subconsciousness, this tyrannical organisation can and will ruthlessly destroy those who fail the obedience and subservience tests, just as easily as it builds up and rewards those subjects more obedient and servile to its tainted requirements.

Orwell's 'Nineteen eighty-four'.

I'm mesmerised, feverishly devouring each page with a chilling sense of disbelief....

THE TEACHER'S CHAIR CREAKS. *He's on his feet. The lesson's over and it's time to head over to the chemistry lab. The fly stops buzzing; the class yawns, scratches, stretches and starts gathering up books and satchels, but I close the worn covers of the book with reluctance, and, despite the heat, with a shiver and a frisson of fear. Such an alien, hostile world that I've just dipped into. Something perhaps all too familiar to millions elsewhere; living suppressed, totalitarian lives under despotic, oppressive state regimes.*

But it's OK.

This is Great Britain. The cradle of democracy, bastion of human dignity and respect, champion of fair justice, honesty, law and order, free universal high-quality healthcare and education, and, of course, global flag carrier for free speech, morality, integrity, honesty, human rights and the unassailable privileges of an open, liberated citizenry.

Not perfect, but as close as any nation has got....

And I silently thank God that I'll never in my lifetime be subject to such dehumanising, state-funded and approved hate and retaliation, brainwashing, lies, and corrupt, destructive and oppressive practices from a huge, ruthless and monopolistic state entity.

PART II

Peter Read's Family's Story
By Karen Read

DAD'S DEATH

NICOLA HAD GONE TO GET the car and I walked slowly down the corridor supporting mum and contemplating the gravity of what had just happened and who we had just lost.

'Mum, I think we need to go and speak to someone about dad's death as I feel once we leave the hospital we won't be able to do anything about it,' I said.

'No I don't want to,' was her reply but after another ten paces she had changed her mind and so we made our back in a bid to speak to someone from the Intensive Care Unit regarding our concerns.

We had just witnessed dad's life slip away after his life support machine had been turned off. It was a truly traumatic day that none of us would ever forget.

That was over six years ago now and sadly, incredulously, and somewhat inexcusably, we still don't have the truth behind dad's avoidable and untimely death. How difficult can it be to get the truth?

Extremely difficult is the answer and, in our experience, it's been near impossible.

Back in May 2015 mum, Nicola and I went to Lancaster Magistrates' Court for dad's inquest. This was a daunting experience for us; we had, of course, never been through anything like this before and we had been given extraordinarily little knowledge of how the procedure was to unfold.

The only kind face we saw on our way into the hearing was that belonging to a gentleman who we knew as Mr Duffy who came over immediately to speak to mum and offer his condolences.

I remember thinking to myself that this was the kind-hearted doctor who mum and I had spoken to outside dad's ward on Boxing

Day 2014; the doctor who had listened intently to our worries and concerns and who, after a short discussion – and while noting there had already been several missed opportunities to do so, including an instance in November 2014 when the wrong theatre had been booked – said he would try to get dad on the theatre list for either Monday the 29th of December or Tuesday the 30th of December in order to get dad's overdue stent changed.

The inquest was our first real ordeal since dad's death – the first opportunity we had to properly address what had gone wrong with his care at the Royal Lancaster Infirmary. A week before the inquest we received copies of various reports and documents which would be presented as evidence and one statement, from Peter Duffy, made incredibly harrowing reading.

In his statement Peter said that, had he been on duty the weekend of the 27th and 28th of December, dad's outcome could have, and in our honest opinion would have, been very different.

We listened, intently and anxiously, during the three-and-a-half-hour inquest, as we tried to take in the detail of the events covering the last few days of dad's life.

The coroner, Ms Hammond, said she wanted to know if there had been any kind of departmental discussion regarding dad's case. Such discussions, which are known as Morbidity and Mortality meetings, are not intended to apportion blame but simply to discuss how, as a team, the urology department might learn from what happened.

The answer, from Mr Duffy, was, to our surprise and dismay – 'no', and so the coroner formally ordered that such a discussion should take place. She instructed that the urology department reflect on the circumstances of dad's death; what happened between the 27th and 29th of December, and for the findings to be reported back to her within six weeks.

The next scheduled Morbidity and Mortality meeting wasn't due to be held for some time and as a result Ms Hammond agreed to an extension of the deadline.

What happened next we only discovered three years later. Following the coroner's order, we had received no update from the hospital and Nicola had spent a lot of time chasing the coroner's office for information.

We eventually discovered, many years later, that the length of time we were subjected to was in fact because two of the three consultants involved in dad's case had refused to discuss the case despite having been instructed to do so by the coroner.

We were told by UHMBT that a root cause analysis (RCA) would take place instead. Although at this time we were informed of the RCA taking place, quite what an RCA was, still remained a mystery to us as did the reasons behind it being completed when the instructions from the coroner seemed to us, extremely clear. However, the RCA did in fact become an integral part of our ongoing story.

Nicola and I were invited to a meeting at Westmoreland General Hospital in October 2015 to discuss the findings of the original RCA. This seemed a difficult and heavy-going meeting but it was nothing compared to what was going to happen over the next five and-a-half years.

After much discussion and an occasional thump of a fist on the table, the then clinical lead eventually admitted that dad's care had not been good. As I remember promises were made that things would change for the better and procedures would follow stronger guidelines. One of these more 'laughable' procedures was a ludicrous invitation for Nicola and me to join the Sepsis panel at the hospital. That is correct; that was what was thought of as a 'good idea' to put two people with absolutely zero medical knowledge on a panel!

Deciding that we could not be bought with this blatant attempt to 'tickle our egos', we politely declined. We were not completely satisfied with the outcome of this meeting; however, it was better than nothing and with reassurances on the points we had raised, improvements would be made.

Nicola and I were relieved. Our mission had been clear to us from the very beginning, we simply wanted no other family or patient to endure the sloppy care that we had unfortunately witnessed and the devastating results this so-called care had ended in.

Result!

Or so we thought. How wrong could we be?

It was a Friday afternoon in August 2018, and I was meeting my dear friend Ann-Marie in town. Whilst putting the world to rights over a cup of tea, Ann-Marie asked if I would accompany her into a particular shop; she had lost a magazine with a CD attached the previous day and wanted some moral support to see if it had been returned.

Casually glancing at the newspapers in the shop there was a face staring at me, a familiar face but one I couldn't quite put a name to. Then the penny dropped…Mr Duffy.

The article from one of our local papers was talking about an avoidable death of a patient in early 2015. I couldn't quite believe what I was seeing or reading, I quickly bought the paper and got out of the shop visibly shaking. I rang Nicola immediately with news that I had something to show her.

Having read the article, we both came to the same conclusion, somehow, we needed to find out if it was actually our dad that Peter was talking about when he mentioned an avoidable death.

Ann-Marie, super sleuth to the rescue, found a telephone number for Mr Duffy on the Isle of Man. Rather than ringing, I sent a text message stating that Nicola and I had read an article in the local paper and were concerned that he might be talking about our father.

My mobile phone rang that evening with the same number; my heart was in my mouth. It was indeed Mr Duffy from the Isle of Man, only it was the wrong Mr Duffy! However after reading my message, he knew it was too important not to respond or reply. I explained my worries, the gentleman told me there was only one hospital on the Island, and to contact Noble's hospital, and that I should be able to track down the correct Mr Duffy.

I now had an email address but had been informed Mr Duffy was on annual leave. I began compiling a detailed account and inquiring if it was our dad that he had been talking about. By 11.30am of the morning of his return to work there a ping to my email inbox with a reply; saying that sadly it was our dad he was referring to and that there had also been a disobedience to the coroner's request.

And so, another three years of hard slog began. I cannot tell you how many emails I have sent, how many phone calls there have been between Nicola and I, or how times I have been asked, 'What do you actually want from all of this?'

Our goal has always been the same, just simply to get the truth about dad's care.

My first job was to write a letter to the Chief Executive of the hospital, Aaron Cummins. First lesson learnt, do not write a letter as they can go missing and you will not get an answer, so I emailed late one Thursday evening. Within five minutes, ping, a reply; immediately with an apology, no letter had made it into his hands. And so began the enormous task of getting our story out to the Trust and avidly trying to ensure that they would actually listen to our concerns. This is no mean feat; you have to be a determined person who is not afraid to be persistent. When it is your flesh and blood and you strongly believe there has been a wrong-doing then you have to stick with it, to right the wrong.

Nicola and I quickly learnt that nothing happens at speed, especially when asking for information and then when you do finally begin to receive paperwork it would sometimes come in so heavily redacted that it was completely impossible to read. Emails started swinging to and fro. Freedom of Information requests, every question opened up more questions and the answers were not always what the family wanted to hear and at times just being totally 'fobbed off'.

After the release of Peter's book, *Whistle in the Wind*, the momentum really picked up another gear. Nicola and I were inundated with messages of support and concern, the press also started to show an interest too.

It was around early September 2019 that Nicola and I had our first meeting face to face with Aaron and the clinical lead that was in charge when dad was in hospital. To say we were nervous was an understatement, but they were both were so lovely and put us at ease. As was to become the normal, I had prepared a speech and questions.

It's exceedingly difficult when you have to talk the talk on medical care using vocabulary that is a complete foreign language to you; give me a ballet class to talk about and I am in my comfort zone, but medical terminology, and hospital protocols can often leave me tongue-tied. Hospital language is full of acronyms which makes it very tricky to understand when you are ploughing through reams and reams of notes, you almost feel you need an interpreter.

It is strange because I am not usually a confident person, but when you are fighting for a loved one an inner strength comes from nowhere, so here we are at the hospital with the Chief Executive and a urology consultant. As Nicola put it, 'there were some toe-curling moments', as I asked countless awkward questions.

I even at one point apologised to the consultant for putting him on the spot in front of his boss. As a result of our meeting, Nicola and I were promised a new RCA to be done from scratch. This was a great stride forward in our opinion as it meant that the Trust obviously felt that there were still unanswered questions regarding dad's care and treatment.

This sadly and unfortunately, and somewhat consistently in this journey, became another empty promise, and although the second RCA made a charade of the original as it was in essence far a more comprehensive report. However, it was flawed from the beginning as there were no new statements taken from the three major consultants involved in dad's case.

In the family's opinion this was a pivotal error as all it was doing was sticking a plaster over the top of the problem and hoping it would heal itself. Nicola and I were once again invited to a meeting, this was to prove our most trying and difficult to date. The three consultants had had their meeting prior to ours and we had briefly seen and spoken to Mr Duffy on his way out who was visibly shaken and quite distressed.

There were eight of us sat round the table the Chief Executive, Medical Director, a professor who had conducted the second RCA, two other consultants who had some dealings with dad and a representative from the Patient Liaison Service (PALS). The first words that came from one of the consultants said that dad's case could quite easily happen again next week within the Trust.

Silence. What on earth had we been fighting for all this time?

Five years had passed since dad's death with sanctions and promises of change, yet here was a highly respected and knowledgeable consultant telling an experienced and well-informed table that nothing at the Trust had altered. This was an unwanted revelation to many around the table and as shocked as Nicola and I were we could not let it get in the way or unsettle our focus for the questions we had worked hard to put together.

It would be so easy to be intimidated by a highly educated audience but if you are passionate and confident in what you believe then you just have to take a deep breath and dive in. It is always such a relief to come out these meetings and feel that some form of progress is being made.

Our next hurdle was to push for the departmental meeting (M&M) which the coroner had requested back in 2015. It was finally going to happen albeit five and a half years late.

Although we were not invited, Nicola and I were extremely disappointed to hear that the usual time for a group discussion was not adhered to and it became more of a presentation rather than a debate, where the whole urology department could use it as a beneficial learning outcome for all involved and would give the family the reassurance that the Trust really did mean to make things better.

I'm not quite sure how it happened but I sent an email asking the Medical Director about the availability of ICU (Intensive Care Unit) beds on Sunday 28th December 2014 and the Trust's protocol when the ICU is full. It was just after the M&M meeting, and I got copied into an email, presumably by mistake. It was asking the now Clinical Lead, who was also one of the three consultants who dealt with dad to reflect on the meeting and consider writing a letter of apology to the family.

Yes, after five and a half years we were expected to believe that a letter that has been asked for by the Medical Director, which consisted of just eight lines, was a sufficient apology. To add insult to injury it completely omitted mum, which Nicola and I found extremely disrespectful. When I questioned this ugly scenario, I was told that it absolutely was a genuine reflection.

Nicola and I did not buy it.

The letter went on to acknowledge the failings in dad's care but failed to be explicit and explain exactly what failings he was talking about and that he and the department had learnt a lot.

So, to sum up in a nutshell, Nicola and I got a letter, five and a half years late after it was asked for by the Medical Director with eight lines apologising for failings. Far too little, far too late.

For the attention of Karen and Nicola (the family of Mr Peter Read)

As part of the consultant team and the wider urology team looking after Mr Read during his last illness, I acknowledge the failings in Mr Peter Reads care surrounding the period from 26.12.14-30.12.2014 and would like to apologise to you all. I also acknowledge the pain and distress this must have caused you all especially due to the time scale and publicity surrounding these issues. I would like to assure that personally and as a department we have learned a lot after reflecting on these failings and the RCA investigation which was conducted. I would also like to assure that these investigations and reflections have brought about changes in our clinical practice to avoid similar incidences occurring in future.

With kind regards
xxxxxxxxxxxxxxxxxxxxxx
Consultant Urological Surgeon
Clinical Lead in Urology
Dated: 8th July 2020

By now the company tasked with carrying out a full investigation into both dad's case and the wider urology department had been appointed. NHS England wanted a full in-depth report. A letter had been sent to Health Secretary signed by four local MP's and the failings at UHMBT had been brought to the attention of parliament.

Niche Health and Social Care Consulting were the company challenged with the unenviable task of sorting out an incredibly entwined and complex series of problems at UHMBT, which had always been reported by their management team as historical. The Terms of Reference were published (TOR).

These were unimportant to Nicola and me; we just wanted the truth. Yes, we are still harping on about that…the truth.

Niche contacted me via email asking if we would be willing to speak and give our account of dad's time in hospital and the events leading up to the present day. This we were only too happy to do and oblige with the evidence we had accumulated and collated and over five and a half years.

Our first face-to-face meeting was 5th March 2020 just as the pandemic was rearing its ugly head. Nicola and I were keen to give our side of dad's story, our concerns and portray the issues that we felt had been neglected and swept under the carpet.

Our meetings were always emotionally draining as the questioning could feel quite intense, purely because of the topic we were speaking about. I often felt that I was in the witness box giving evidence at a trial.

From the very beginning, our story has never changed simply because it was and is the truth. As the Niche report of dad's case was coming to an end, Nicola and I were assigned a psychologist. We thought this was rather alarming but with hindsight it was a great decision as we were to discover.

The draft report was released to about 14 people who had to sign a Non-Disclosure Agreement (NDA) to have access to the document. They were given 14 days to reply with their feedback, concerns, inaccuracies, and questions. Once they were in, then Nicola and I were able to read the document. We did not sign an NDA but were encouraged not to speak to the press or any journalists as Niche did not want any part of the report being leaked out to the public.

Dad's report was 148 pages long. Reading it from cover to cover for the first time was so emotionally draining. Sometimes if you watch a film or read a book over and over you might live in hope that the ending will change, and everyone lives happily ever after. Reading this report was like being back at the hospital just over six years ago but the outcome, the story's ending was not going to change; and it was heart-breaking.

Our psychologist gave us excellent advice on how to break up the report and absorb the information piece by piece. There were 46 recommendations under nine specific categories, which explains to even ordinary people, like Nicola and I, how severe the problems were at UHMBT.

Together, with the psychologist, we worked through the report. He helped us decipher difficult and complicated medical jargon and at times challenged us on our thoughts and reasoning as more questions came to the forefront of our minds. A final piece of work was to be done by Nicola and me, before the report could be completed and sent to NHS England. A challenge if ever there was for the grieving family.

A Family Statement was required to go at the front of the report. This was to paint a picture of dad, his life and how his death had affected mum, Nicola, myself, and the rest of the family. A daunting task and one that I was reluctant and unsure quite where to start. However, our psychologist gave us a list of questions to work through as a starting point and as if by magic the daunting job became much easier to handle.

Our Family Statement.

Dad was born in 1939 in Catford and was lucky enough to attend Dulwich College. From there he went into the Merchant Navy serving as an Officer for the Blue Funnel Line, sailing all over the world. It was whilst he was in the port of Liverpool that he met mum at the Jacaranda Club. They were married 1.12.1962 and celebrated their Golden Wedding in 2012.

Dad continued to serve in the Merchant Navy until he got a job in Heysham working for Sealink and the family moved to More- cambe in 1967. Dad worked his way up to Captain before becoming the Port Manager at Heysham. Dad brought the dying port back on its feet and was the instigator of the port's resurgence. He was ex- tremely well respected with all the workers from the dockers to company managers who did business with the port. He worked there until he retired in 1998.

We never knew how dad was going to fill his time when he re-tired as he was married to his job, but mum soon became a golf widow. Holidays and travelling all over the world with friends became mum and dad's focus for well-deserved enjoyment time together. They built a spectacular list of enviable places to visit and indulged in many hours planning and discussing their next desti-nation. I once asked dad if there was one place in the world he would tell us to visit where would it be, his answer very swiftly was Bali.

Dad was never idle, there was always a structure to the day. He could turn his hand pretty much to anything and there was nothing he liked more than pottering around in the garden, which he kept immaculate.

Nicola and I could always ask for help and advice with any-thing, and he would be there like a shot, in the garden expertly cutting the lawn, mending fences, tidying and of course lots of invaluable life skills guidance. As children we had a happy child-hood with holidays and activities, friends over to stay but when dad said 'No' you knew not to ask again.

Dad started to have some health issues around 2009, but this never stopped him from enjoying life. You never heard him com-plain and he was still playing golf up until October 2014.

It was a great testament to dad how well he was both respected and thought of by friends and colleagues from across the country, as his funeral was packed to capacity. There was standing room only and the doors were left open for people to stand out in the corridor and pay their respects.

Dad's death has rocked the entire family to the core, especially our mum, who, although she is a strong character, has been totally lost without her soul mate, and it has taken its toll in her confi-dence. Mum had been through every step with dad during his illness and had visited him relentlessly every day whilst in hospital, and most days twice daily. Mum and dad were both of the genera-tion that did not want any fuss making for fear of 'rocking the boat'. Questions regarding dad's care were for the doctors and not for the family to query. There is now a great void in mum's life. Nicola and I have lost our Jiminy Cricket who was always there with wise words: 'If you can't say something nice then don't say anything'.

Dad had fought his cancer with courage and fortitude and was making an exceptional recovery, looking forward to the future and better times ahead but this was not to be because of a catalogue of dire missed opportunities, dreadful decisions, poor and inadequate management and a basic lack of human care, kindness and thought for others. Fundamental requirements for any Hospital Trust.

This has been made worse due to the six year struggle the family have had to endure in trying to establish the full truth, this has been like getting blood out of a stone. The whole process has been filled with lies, deceit and what has felt to us like one big cover up with no one wanting to take ownership for the wrongs that most definitely have been done.

In our view, from reading the report we acknowledge that there were far too many missed opportunities in which both dad's treatment and care could have been massively improved. There can be differences of opinions between medical professionals, and we accept that mistakes can be made, but we are also painfully aware that hindsight is more of an exact science.

However, we feel that given the obvious decline in dad over the entirety of his last admission, the critical tipping point was the blood results which arrived in the early morning hours of the 27th December 2014. It is therefore incomprehensible to us that that dad was not taken to theatre sooner, especially as it became apparent that the antibiotics he was given for the onset of sepsis were not taking effect and dad was slipping away before our very eyes.

We, the family, have always been led to believe that this was an isolated incident but from media coverage we now know that this was far from the case. There have been patients and families that have suffered unnecessarily through sloppy urological care and a management that failed to listen. Dad's case was entirely predictable.

We have been through not only the grieving process of losing our loved one (husband, father, grandad, great grandad) but have also endured an inquest, two Root Cause Analyses and an Independent Inquiry together with many meetings at the hospital with the Chief Executive, Medical Director, Consultants, Professors and many other, all of which have taken their toll.

My sister and I have done this solely by ourselves, in which we have spent a great many hours of researching all manner of medical and governance issues which is extremely difficult when you have no prior knowledge. Each time we have an episode and think we are there, then something else rears its ugly head and we are off again. Mum has not been involved in any of the procedures since the Inquest as she said it was too distressing for her and none of this would bring dad back.

Since the Niche Report has been out, both Nicola and I have been seeing a psychologist to help us understand our feelings and help us come to terms with our loss and the emotional rollercoaster over the past six years. Nicola and I have continued our quest in the hopes that this disgraceful and toxic environment can be sorted once and for all and that no other patient and their family has to suffer cruel and needless heartache that we the Read family have been subjected to.

A hospital should be a safe and caring place to send a loved one.

The Family Statement complete, another couple of recommendations that Nicola and I felt needed adding to the report and some questions that we had regarding the section headed 'Final episode of care' the psychologist then asked if we were ready for a final meeting with Niche? 'Yes please'.

Our final meeting with Niche to tie up loose ends, before dad's report was due to go to NHS England was just awful. Nicola and I came off the Teams meeting of three hours and forty minutes totally traumatised and unable to understand what had gone so terribly wrong.

As per usual, I had written an opening statement thanking Niche for all their hard work and the detailed account of dad's care from UHMBT they had uncovered. We also personally thanked each person individually who had always shown us the utmost compassion, care and thoughtfulness and continually sent kind words to mum.

I then went on to say that in our opinion when looking at dad's case as a stand out case it seemed to take some issues out of context, the bigger picture needed to be looked at to paint a true reflection of dad's story.

Dad's report did not touch on the cultural problems within the urology department. However, this played a huge part in dad's case. Had management been strong from the beginning and not turned a blind eye, refusing to see the ever spiralling out of control problems and tackling them with a strong leadership as one would expect from a national institution from the start, possibly going back as far as 2010 at UHMBT, then just maybe a diverse cultural department could have worked in harmony rather than working in discord with consultants working in fear of a racism allegation being brought against them for speaking up against poor and dangerous working practises, as we have read in *Whistle in the Wind*.

Our problems started in earnest as soon as I finished reading the Family Statement, which I was secretly proud of. Firstly, it was deemed too long and then there were too many negative adjectives! What were we supposed to do here? Paint a picture of butterflies and rainbows?!

I pointed out that I had only followed the psychologist's questions to help navigate and produce the piece and as far as negative adjectives were concerned having ploughed through 148 pages of cynical report writing there was nothing positive to say. The psychologist was quick to jump to our defence and put a powerful case forward and justifying our words. Time for reflection was asked for by the team to consider our words.

The next major issue concerned Mr Duffy. It became increasingly clear to both Nicola and me that Mr Duffy was coming under constant and unnecessary fire.

It is true to say that Niche have been extremely uncomfortable with the fact that we had any dialogue with Peter over the last three years and this was not 'professional' in their opinion. This has always seemed ludicrous to us as we are firmly all on the same side and that side is the safety and well-being of all patients who cross the threshold of a hospital to be cared for in a safe, protected, and steadfast manner befitting an institution such as the NHS.

I spoke up and out with much frustration regarding the excessive and pointed way that the meeting was being constantly drawn back to Mr Duffy, in an effort, it seemed to us, to place the blame firmly at his feet.

Every time I asked a question relating to decisions made or not made (despite factual medical readings and advice from a microbiologist), on the 27th December the repetitive reply that came was 'Well if Mr Duffy on the 26th December had just....' This was so blatantly unjust. It was even suggested to us during the meeting that 'Mr Duffy was probably able to shout louder than other consultants' and therefore able get dad into theatre when needed.

If Mr Duffy had had a crystal ball on the 26th December, then maybe circumstances would have been different. Other consultants had reference to screaming blood results early on the 27th December which should have been acted upon immediately, and in the family's opinion was the crucial tipping point. Had dad been given swift medical attention, who knows what the outcome may have been. It is true to say that the family were significantly surprised by the description used by Niche to portray the lack of action over a very sick patient. It was referred to as a *'lack of curiosity...'*

Really?!

The meeting left Nicola and me in a full-blown state of shock as we both felt distraught and totally intimidated. It was not how we believed any grieving family should be treated. We had always been so willing and fully cooperative throughout the whole process, after all, we just wanted the truth not spin where the easiest route was to blame the whistleblower, rather than deal with the enormous sinkhole that seems to be getting bigger with every turning of a blind eye.

This whole experience has been traumatic from the start. Nicola and I have been asked numerous times what we want from it all and the answer is simply, the truth. But that is unlikely to ever happen, until top level management are strong and robust enough to have measures in place to eradicate poor and shoddy system failures that encourage a tiny minority to flagrantly abuse their power to avoid following protocols and procedures thus ensuring a safe and confident place to work, learn and thrive.

Mr Duffy has always and without exception been professional and caring throughout the whole time of this tragic journey from our first meeting on the 26th December 2014 to the present day. I have never been a puppet to say words or ask questions that have come from his mouth. Yes, we have been helped to understand medical terminology and I have occasionally asked for advice but his unwavering belief to speak out and whistle blow for the rights of his patients and their families is relentless and truly humbling.

It has been suggested to us that perhaps Mr Duffy should have kept a professional distance from my sister and me. This I could never understand, as we are all supposed to be singing from the same hymn sheet, trying to get to the truth and prevent poor practises happening in any ward in any hospital and, as the meaning in the dictionary says, the Hippocratic Oath is a promise made by people when they become doctors to do everything possible to help their patients and to have high moral standards in their work.

Nowhere anywhere in the world would you find a more dedicated, kind-hearted, and down to earth consultant who would put everything on the line including his family life for honesty and truth as Mr Duffy.

Karen Read, on behalf of Karen and Nicola.

PART III

The rankest compound of villainous smell that ever offended nostril

The Merry Wives of Windsor (Act 3, Scene 5)

INTRODUCTION

Legion of Failures

•

In 2001, William, our third son was born. We purchased a dream house just down the road from the Royal Lancaster Infirmary and I settled into what seemed to be the perfect life with Fiona and our young family. Despite early struggles...we soon came to love it and it proved the perfect place for our family to grow up....

My parents and old school friends were one stop down the motorway, we were surrounded by farming relatives, I was doing the job that I loved and felt a true vocation for and it seemed that life just couldn't get any better.

Whistle in the Wind (chapter 6, page 29).

ALMOST EXACTLY TWO DECADES ON, this seemingly limitless promise, happiness, attainment and future potential came within a split second of the most abrupt, shocking, corrupt and brutal end imaginable. A smashed and mutilated corpse, broken physically and mentally, crushed into the road surface of a cold, dark and dank alleyway in a small coastal village and fishing port on the west coast of the Isle of Man. A scene utterly redolent with self-loathing, failure and defeat. An individual ensnared and hopelessly trapped in disgrace; their entire adult achievements demeaned, disfigured and destroyed. And, in their mind, facing possible prosecution, disgrace and even incarceration. Alone, distraught and isolated, and with the last vestiges of hope and self-respect brutally cast adrift and comprehensively smashed on the stormy rocks of what ultimately proved to be utterly false, fabricated and backdated email evidence....

Another avoidable death.

After four decades of hard graft, devotion and vocation, following and, to the best of my ability, attempting to exceed every required professional, regulatory and employment standard required of me, and with such an implacable, unshakeable commitment to and belief in NHS standards, how was it possible that I could have been dragged down to such unspeakable depths from those evocative and heady early days of so much latent promise? Degraded, deceived and destroyed by the very state monopoly that I had committed my adult life to serving. A state monopoly that had made such unequivocal promises that acts of governmental and corporate hatred, cruelty, bullying and harassment towards whistleblowers would never happen again.

Caught, and ultimately crushed in the clash between two implacably opposed healthcare forces.

On one hand, the public, shrill, mandatory and unstoppable force of political, organisational, ministerial and regulatory whistleblowing propaganda and posturing, with copious and nauseating quantities of virtue-signalling about candour, safeguarding, honesty and openness.

Yet, on the other hand, the immoveable object of private, covert and corrupt organisational secrecy, spin, false promises, bullying, fear, hatred, cover-ups, betrayals and reputation protection.

––––––––––––

WHISTLE IN THE WIND tried hard to put the circumstances of my whistleblowing and subsequent illegal dismissal into the broader perspective of organisational, regulatory and legal failures. Two years on from publication, and in the context of what is clearly an ongoing, very personal, bitter and, if it were possible, even more brutal, hate-filled and vengeful witch-hunt, it is worth revisiting the legion of failures that chart out the events of the last two decades. In Part III of this latest manuscript, we can, perhaps, fill in some of the gaps left by the broad-brush comments and criticisms made in the conclusions of *Whistle in the Wind* and perhaps, just maybe, try and ensure that something good comes of this whole corrupt and rotten corporate, regulatory and legal disarray.

———————

ON THE FACE OF IT, there are so very many layers of protection on offer to the vulnerable and abused whistleblower, and indeed protections for patients and the general public from poor or inappropriate services or care. However, it is a medical and surgical truism that, where you see a myriad of different treatments and solutions for the same underlying health problem, you can be assured that none of them work very well.

It is no different with whistleblowing and safeguarding.

Organisations produce earnest, sincere and unequivocal promises of whistleblower protection, solemnly and repeatedly pledging no detriment or dismissal to any whistleblowing staff. Regulators like the CQC and GMC play up and, in some cases mandate the act of safeguarding, clearly implying that, by any rational extension of common sense, victimised whistleblowers can reasonably and logically expect substantial and robust regulatory support. On behalf of the state, ministers and senior politicians posture, pledge, preach and promise about *freedom to speak up* and whistleblower legal safeguards. Within the health system itself, a national whistleblower *Guardian* infers the presence of a substantive, powerful personality who will robustly defend, protect and *guard* the beleaguered whistleblower, whilst further additional local guardians exist, putatively to keep their regional NHS organisations in check and accountable. And, of course, the judiciary and senior politicians play up the protections offered by the Public Interest Disclosure Act.

In the meantime, relevant data, evidential and documentary integrity and unfettered access will be protected and secured by civil law, national protocols and the Data Protection Act, according to the mandatory legal requirements of evidential preservation as detailed in Part I, chapter 14. The Freedom of Information Act also creates a public 'right of access' to information held by public authorities, ensuring that such authorities cannot legally withhold any information, particularly that which might be detrimental to public safety.

The legal system itself, we are told, sets the highest standards, with a mandatory requirement that all evidence should be truthfully and honestly disclosed, with substantial penalties threatened (but virtually never carried through) for individuals and organisations which might seek to withhold, distort or fabricate the truth, interfere with witnesses, tamper with or destroy potentially relevant evidence. The courts themselves have made it clear that the standard of honesty required for solicitors and legal professionals is so high as to ensure that they may be *trusted to the ends of the earth* (Bolton v Law Society 1993). Just as the GMC holds the medical profession to account in order to enforce the highest standards, so the legal profession is supposedly held to these similarly high standards by the Solicitors Regulation Authority (SRA).

The Equality and Human Rights Commission polices and enforces the wellbeing of the nation's citizens, ensuring that human rights are not violated, either by the state or by organisations, and guaranteeing equality for all, protecting each and every citizen from acts of hate, prejudice, harassment or discrimination.

Over and above this, and within the public services themselves, the Nolan principles unequivocally commit all public bodies, in addition to the above proscriptions, to show integrity, selflessness, objectivity, leadership, accountability, openness and honesty. These are not negotiable but are the core and mandatory principles that govern the conduct of any public organisation.

And, of course, central to all of this grand discourse is the National Health Service itself.

The impressive sounding NHS Constitution pledges and legally binds the NHS to bringing the highest levels of knowledge, skill and professionalism to save lives and improve health, having a duty to each and every individual that it serves, and respecting their human rights. Aspiring to the highest standards of excellence and professionalism, it commits to providing high quality care that is safe, effective and focused on patient experience. Respect, dignity, compassion and care, we are assured, will be at the core of how patients and staff are treated. Public funds will be devoted solely to the benefit of the people that the NHS serves.

The NHS is, we are told, entirely accountable and transparent to the public, communities and the law, fully committed to speaking up when things go wrong and equally committed to honesty and openness, welcoming feedback from patients, families, carers, and staff, ensuring that compassion is central to the care provided, cherishing excellence and professionalism wherever it is found.

Patients, families, carers and staff will, we are repeatedly assured, be treated with dignity and respect, and will be protected from abuse and neglect, ensuring that the organisation learns lessons from complaints and claims and uses these to improve NHS services.

Additionally, all staff will have rewarding, worthwhile jobs, trusted, actively listened to and provided with meaningful feedback. Respected at work, with fair pay, healthy and safe working conditions and an environment free from harassment, cruelty, bullying or violence, and of course being freely able to raise any concern with their employer, whether it is about safety, malpractice or other risks to general public.

SO WHERE AND HOW, in this colossal glut of grand promises, pledges and assurances; pretty much all of which have been quite openly violated and betrayed, has it all gone so horribly, terribly wrong?

How have we ended up in what, from my perspective, is a parallel, dystopian universe of bullying and abuse, outright prejudice, forced resignations, avoidable deaths and avoidable harm, regulatory blindness, witness intimidation, contempt for the coronial system and indeed for the legal employment tribunal process? Admixed, of course, with threats, lies, retaliation and harassment, broken promises and pledges, evidential spoliation and destruction, blatant inconsistencies in sworn evidence, psychological manipulation, misleading statements, hypocrisy, cover-ups and covert briefings?

We seem to be a million light years away from the utopian world of the ideals listed above.

The rankest compound of villainous smell that ever offended nostril.

What lessons can the NHS, regulators, guardians, ministers, executives, civil servants and the Department of Health draw from my and my family's experiences? And how might we make a start on putting this *legion of failures* right?

CHAPTER ONE

The NHS
Lessons Eternally Unlearned

AS A LEARNING EXPERIENCE it is worth turning the clock back through 15 years and the events of *Whistle in the Wind* and teasing out the myriad of errors that were made along the way. Just possibly, such a distasteful and unsettling exercise might help to inform future administrations as to how to finally break this endless cycle of poor care, patient harms, abuse and cover-up.

Concerns about behaviour from one individual in the UHMBT urology department had already been voiced before I was even appointed in 2000. By 2004, it was clear that, in respect of this individual, we had a major and persisting safety issue, not just with clinical standards and behaviour, but with insight too. After all, who could take twelve targeted prostate biopsies to diagnose a possible cancer, aiming to rigorously sample each at-risk area of the prostate, miss the prostate entirely each and every time, sending only bits of fat and bowel wall to the laboratory, and yet continue to believe that all was well, their technique was beyond reproach and that the prostate had been adequately sampled? Or leave a patient with rapidly progressive and imminently fatal 'flesh-eating' necrotising fasciitis for nearly twenty hours without attention (*Whistle in the Wind*, page 32)? With all the other issues and clinical problems detailed in the earlier publication, there was a massive and potentially lethal issue, not just with technique and training, but with self-awareness and self-scrutiny too, and a desperately urgent need to protect the public from other potentially deadly deviations from the normal.

Yet after years of dithering, with these safety-critical issues finally becoming public (and having been told that I'd have been sacked 18 months earlier if my behaviour had been the same), I was informed, and with pinpoint accuracy, of what the knee-jerk response would be:

Retraining is the answer. Now what's the question?

Retraining is not, of course, the universal answer. Nevertheless, the NHS seems to persist in believing that almost any problem involving dangerous standards and behaviour by senior and difficult-to-dismiss staff can be addressed by retraining, whilst declining to acknowledge that elephant in the room – the fact that, regrettably, it is perfectly possible for some individuals to get all the way to senior and authoritative clinical practice in the NHS whilst being entirely and intrinsically unsuited to such privilege and responsibility.

The correct response should have been to acknowledge the dangerous lack of insight, remove the individual in question from front-line care; protect patients (and in the process protect whistleblowing staff from counter-allegations), ensure that the correct clinical and professional standards were being adhered to within the rest of the department, and find that individual an alternative role which did not involve clinical responsibility and which, above all else, enabled good clinical care to go on without being compromised.

To their credit, I was informed at the time that the Royal College of Surgeons had refused to arrange a retraining programme for the individual in question, responding to requests by pointing out that the issues around lack of insight were serious enough that retraining was clearly not the answer.

Nevertheless, UHMBT clearly knew better, and by reportedly allowing the surgeon in question to arrange their own retraining programme, thereby firmly set the department on the road to chaos and anarchy, in the process both wrecking and taking several lives, and the careers and prospects of several others.

I too ought to take responsibility for a major failing at this point. Agonising over whether to approach the GMC over my concerns, I was sufficiently fearful both of counter-allegations and the conventional fate of NHS whistleblowers to decide against this, reassuring myself that I'd done the right thing in flagging up concerns internally and could better serve my patients by keeping my job and an otherwise low profile, rather than approach a regulator and end up unemployed and potentially even unemployable.

It was, undoubtedly, a bad mistake. Had I plucked up sufficient courage to definitively approach my regulator much earlier, the outcomes for myself, colleagues, patients and relatives might have been significantly better.

In my defence, it is, of course, highly likely that I would simply have found myself demoted, defrauded, disciplined and dismissed a decade earlier....

Compounding my and the NHS's mistakes, UHMBT, upon the completion of retraining, insisted upon secrecy rather than openness. *Nothing to be in writing. Any concerns to be expressed by word of mouth and behind closed doors only....* Of course, this simply embeds further a culture of fear and cover-up, discourages whistleblowing and encourages the errant individual who triggered the concerns to believe that they have the upper hand.

With the truly tragic and avoidable death of Mrs Irene Erhart at Furness General Hospital in 2011, internal UHMBT alarm bells should have been ringing hysterically. Failure to act and take responsibility over a deteriorating patient by two consultant surgeons was bad enough. But ward nursing staff having to request that a third surgeon be called over to take charge in an urgent, deteriorating and potentially life-threatening case, despite that third party surgeon being based nearly 50 miles away, having nothing to do with the case, no presence or timetabled activities at the hospital in question and having to attend to the case in their spare time is, to the best of my knowledge, unheard of.

Clearly, retraining had failed abysmally, a patient's life, yet again, was critically endangered and now, self-evidently, poor practice and inappropriate attitudes had spread further within the department. Yet, when it all ended in disaster, and despite a subsequent, damning coroner's verdict, precisely nothing happened. The moratorium on written comments and expressions of concern about dangerous practice remained and standards continued unchanged, jeopardising more lives and causing yet more disquiet and disharmony in the department.

2014 to 2015, as documented in *Whistle in the Wind*, ended with yet more errors, neglect and, of course, another avoidable death. By this point, UHMBT were very well aware of the fact that there were towering issues of clinical safety amongst a very small number in the department. Yet, despite overwhelming evidence of poor practice, risk taking and neglect, executives seemed to prefer to regard the issues as a *dysfunctional department*, rather than asking the rather more awkward but far more relevant question of why such serious errors kept occurring. And how a department that, in around 2008 was winning public plaudits, awards and national recognition for the quality, efficiency, innovation and consistency of its care was, suddenly and within just a few years, generating attention for all the wrong reasons.

Responding, instead by glossing over the clinical failings and instead organising a psychological review of the department (something that was entirely unnecessary and inappropriate for 90% of the department), UHMBT's management completely failed to act upon the fact that the rapidly fragmenting department was a clear consequence of repeated lapses in standards from a small number of consultants, preferring the much more convenient group-blame explanation of childish, immature staff who cannot get on together.

Nowhere is weak corporate and investigative leadership more evident than in the frequent dismissal of internal whistleblowing disputes as a *dysfunctional department*. Used as a common, if not ubiquitous excuse for inaction over speaking up, safeguarding and the inevitable counter-allegations, this lazy phrase implies childish behaviour, a general falling-out and failures to relate to each other.

Children quarrelling in a playground and *personality clashes*. Thus, it is possible to divert attention away from the clinical errors and omissions, the candour and whistleblowing, together with the associated retaliation and counter-allegations and simplify the issue into one of inadequate personalities; thereby absolving executives and managers of any accountability for their failure to protect patients and address the underlying problem of poor outcomes.

After all, it's a *dysfunctional department* isn't it? Weak characters and poor self-discipline.

Everyone's and no one's fault and, of course, a major insult to those decent, hardworking staff who are simply trying to speak up, protect and improve the service and safeguard vulnerable patients and other employees.

Even a single utterance of the phrase *dysfunctional department* in the context of failing safety standards should immediately mandate the asking of the question – *why?*

What was the trigger for the *dysfunctionality?*

In the case of the urology department, the Medical Director of UHMBT himself openly conceded that it was *Mr A, Mr B and Mr Madhra on one side, and everyone else on the other....* Yet there seemed a complete and astonishing lack of any curiosity as to how such a division might have arisen, or whether clearly sincere and longstanding expressions of concern on one side over clinical, personal and professional behaviour, originating from patients and staff both within and without the urology department, and counter-allegations of bullying, racism and prejudice on the other carried the weight of any evidence behind them. Even a cursory glance would have demonstrated that there was overwhelming evidence to back up the former concerns, and none whatsoever to substantiate the latter. Indeed, the very same UHMBT Medical Director also conceded that, in relation to the counter-allegations of abuse, racism and prejudice, the NHS had *never found anything actionable.*

But how much easier it is to simply label the problems as a *dysfunctional department* and turn the blame, at least in part, back onto the whistleblowers themselves....

Early 2015 was yet another major missed opportunity for UHMBT to decisively and courageously intervene on behalf of the patients and staff. Another avoidable death, two high-profile resignations and a bullying and abusive phone call – a witnessed call which very nearly resulted in a third resignation too. A situation only remedied with my removal to the other side of the Trust. Yet, once again, the further disintegration of the department and loss of valued staff along the fault lines of clinical and professional standards seemed to trigger no meaningful executive response, where it should have merited immediate intervention. Instead, there was, once again, a sense of corporate helplessness and rudderlessness over the frankly dangerous behaviour going on right under their noses.

Summer of 2015 represented another new low, with an arrogant act of outright disobedience to the coroner's court, in an ultimately successful attempt to defy Ms Hammond's orders, prevent open, candid departmental discussion and learning in respect of the second avoidable death case, and block the departmental consensus from being passed back to the coroner's office as we had been formally instructed to do. Yet the response, once again, was entirely wrong, with a complete failure to back up and enforce the coroner's order and an equally abject and miserable failure to sanction those who had shown such contempt for the coroner's legal authority. This was followed, shortly after, by a hopelessly inadequate Root Cause Analysis report as an alternative to complying with Ms Hammond's order and obeying her instructions to obtain a departmental consensus. Even when HM coroner rejected the report; threatening a regulation 28[11] over the issues in the department (see *Whistle in the Wind*, chapter 12), no meaningful action was taken, the RCA report in question remaining on the record for another four to five years, purporting to be an accurate, impartial and faithful representation of events when the reality couldn't have been more different.

By this point and with ongoing clinical and surgical risk-taking, I had involved the Care Quality Commission (CQC). Yet over a period of nearly 12 months, quite unbelievably, no attempt whatsoever was

---

[11] A formal and public Notification of Risk to the Public by the coroner.

made by the CQC to contact, interview or meet up with any of the other members of the department to corroborate and triangulate my concerns and see if my anxieties were shared by others. Nor was any attempt made by UHMBT to properly inform the CQC and ask for assistance over a situation that was clearly continuing to deteriorate. Had the Trust done so, the CQC would have been left in no doubt about the risks to both patients and staff, but once more, apathy, inaction and poor leadership reigned.

I must again take my share of responsibility for the failings and cover-up at this point. Once the CQC's entirely flaccid position on these failings became clear, I really should have forcefully approached the General Medical Council and stuck with this approach, rather than initially discussing my fears with them and then withdrawing such concerns over the fear of revenge and retaliatory allegations. Instead, I clung on to the hope that the CQC's dithering and inaction would eventually firm up into something more robust.

It was not to be.

There was, at this point, yet another major missed opportunity. Mr John Dickinson (our surgical associate specialist) and I stood for the interim departmental lead post in late 2015, making the issue of departmental, clinical and professional standards and the safety of patients the central pillar of our philosophy. An extract from my letter of application is provided in *Whistle in the Wind*, page 120 and made, I hope, a powerful point of highlighting the failing standards and behaviour in a small part of the department and the need for urgent change. Jointly appointed, this was, I believe, a last opportunity for UHMBT's executive to throw their weight behind John, myself and the large majority of the department, try and turn the situation around from within the organisation and demand new and uniformly high standards of personal and professional behaviour from everyone.

John and I had made it clear that we were prepared to directly suffer the backlash and brickbats of taking a stand on these issues but would need heavyweight corporate support. Yet, in the end UHMBT's senior management bottled it, instead allowing the covert campaign of retaliatory allegations to gather further momentum, and, under pressure, demoting both myself and John just months later in early 2016, just as we hoped and believed that we were starting to make a real difference.

It was a truly massive failure of corporate courage, governance and leadership.

After taking a defining stand on personal and professional standards within the department, attracting an immediate push-back from those small number in the department and the wider Trust who were unhappy with such a new direction and, having refused to be silenced about poor behaviour and clinical concerns, a number of potentially illegal and punitive actions rapidly followed; all driven by the Critical Care Division of UHMBT, all clearly formulated to weaken my grip on the job and all of them being well known corporate tactics used against errant whistleblowers (see *Postscript*). The retaliation culminated, not only in a refusal by UHMBT to refund the five-figure sum deducted from my salary, but also in a not-very-veiled-at-all threat to go back through my previous years of earnings *recouping monies*.

It is difficult to contemplate a greater act of corporate bullying and abuse. Yet the executives of UHMBT remained mute and seemingly comfortable with such clear abuses of employment law. The entire board and HR department, despite their unequivocal whistleblower protection promises and pledges, did precisely nothing except, of course, to quietly airbrush out such corporate promises a couple of years later as the employment tribunal date approached. Furthermore, the new departmental lead who replaced John and myself, together with the divisional managers and divisional lead clinician, the Medical Director, executives, non-executives and whistleblower guardian should have been all over such a grotesque act of bullying, illegal whistleblower retaliation, prejudice and illegal breaches of employment law.

Yet silence prevailed.

Summer of 2016 was, in my opinion, another period of craven spinelessness and absent leadership. Forced into resignation by the significant and growing sums of money pillaged from my earnings, and facing the overt threat of a retrospective and clearly illegal further raid on the family finances, there was no possible alternative but to rapidly work out my notice, separate myself from such corporate and organisational prejudice as quickly as I could and join the ranks of the unemployed. This cannot possibly have gone unnoticed by senior managers, executives and non-executives; particularly as, in an intensely surreal moment, I'd just picked up their UHMBT *Doctor of the Year* Award. Yet not one single member of the medical hierarchy or Trust executive had the courage, morals, leadership abilities and conviction to involve themselves in my case, preferring instead to hide behind the high walls of the corporate NHS fortress, declining even any face-to-face meetings until my notice was worked out and my UHMBT and NHS career over.

The CQC were equally keen to wash their hands of me. We had one face-to-face meeting in late 2016 where I provided detailed accounts to several CQC senior managers, both in relation to clinical standards and my brutal illegal dismissal. Despite expressions of shock, things went precisely no further. Even during the regular meetings between the CQC and UHMBT executives, no attempt was made to hold UHMBT's board to their promises of whistleblower protection and, by early 2017, I'd given up on the CQC too.

Not only had UHMBT flagrantly violated and betrayed their own board's promises and assurances, they'd also shamelessly repeated once again the errors, misjudgements, poor leadership and cover-ups of the midwifery scandal, in itself a catastrophic series of executive errors that senior UHMBT executives had repeatedly pledged in front of the national media would never, ever happen again.

CHAPTER TWO

The Regulators

SO VERY MUCH IS made of regulatory protection for whistleblowers and yet there is so very little substance behind it. It is another axiom that human beings always tend to take the easy way out of any decision or conundrum, and nowhere is this more true than for those who find themselves in positions of power and authority. In the regulatory organisations, the buck-passing and abdications of responsibility reach whole new levels, almost becoming an art form in themselves.

With UHMBT having miserably failed to clear a public protection and corporate standards bar that was set so low that it was almost subterranean, a whole series of entirely ineffective and craven external regulators also managed to stumble and face-plant over this hurdle too. Numerous authorities were approached, by telephone, letter and email for support in the aftermath of my unashamedly illegal dismissal. Each and every one obeyed the *route of least resistance* rule, and either declined to take on my case, or passed the issue on to someone else. Trying to get any single regulator to fulfil their obligations, show leadership and courage, take ownership and responsibility, get involved on the side of the whistleblower and, of course, the at-risk public was about as productive as trying to fit shoes on a snake.

Thus, the CQC simply accepted UHMBT's platitudes and assurances, determinedly looking the other way whilst my job and career was systematically destroyed, claiming that it wasn't able to get involved in employment disputes, no matter how illegal.

Of course, each and every one of us can get involved in opposing illegal or corrupt activity. The CQC's position is, perhaps, analogous to a road traffic police officer looking the other way during a mugging and then claiming to have been unable to get involved on the basis that there was no driving violation.

The GMC seemingly learned nothing from the Hooper report of 2015,[12] accepting, in late 2019, a barrage of ridiculous allegations against myself despite their clear retaliatory nature and complete lack of any evidential background, dragging the whole stressful investigative process out over some 15 months.

The National Guardian's Office (responsible for overseeing the *Freedom to Speak Up* campaign within the NHS) repeatedly refused to get involved, citing the ongoing possibility of litigation. Of course, once the litigation was over, the excuse became that the case was now historical and time expired.

Attending a 2018 whistleblowing meeting in London, the head of the National Guardian's Office epitomised the attitude of so many state regulators by disengaging herself from conversation with me within a few seconds of realising who I was, turning her back, beating a hurried retreat and hastily striking up a conversation on the other side of the room.

Having reported the episode of contempt of court and disobedience to the coroner to the Attorney General's office and, despite providing them with clear proof of the act of disobedience (see *Whistle in the Wind*, chapter 11) I was informed that the evidential burden required to take such a case further was high, and therefore not worth pursuing, despite the presence of an avoidable death at the centre of the case. Yet there was clear, unequivocal proof of such an act of contempt, both in the emails of the time and the fact that, self-evidently, the coroner's orders that were witnessed by the coroner's officer and the entire bereaved family had gone unfulfilled for some five years.

Clearly, even hard proof is insufficient to pursue a contempt of court case and one can only speculate on what level of disaster

---

[12] https://www.gmc-uk.org/-/media/documents/ Hooper_review_final_60267393.pdf.

would have to happen to jerk the Attorney General's office out of their torpor and encourage them to protect public safety by enforcing the primacy of UK and coroner's court orders.

Astonishingly, the local senior coroner responded to my attempts to buttress and support the primacy of the coroner's court and coronial orders by making it clear in robust, if not rude terms, that any further communications from me would be deleted or binned.

The Solicitors Regulation Authority dragged things out with, essentially, no action for some twelve months before assuring me that UHMBT and their legal team's actions in threatening costs and intimidating the main witness (whilst all the time withholding vital witness and written evidence and knowing that their own case was fatally undermined by evidential concealment, destruction and a pivotal piece of evidence that they'd had declared as sub-judice), was all, in the SRA's opinion, perfectly acceptable legal behaviour and entirely reasonable in a UK court of law.

THE OTHER REGULATORS, over both emails and telephone conversations, proved equally flaccid, as described in *Whistle in the Wind*.

NHS England initially showed some interest, but finally decided that they were only responsible for community care and standards in General Practice, telling me over the 'phone that Foundation Trusts were independent and NHS England was therefore unable to intervene.

NHS Improvement dithered, and finally referred the case back to the CQC who had, of course, already washed their hands of me.

The Equality and Human Rights Commission excused themselves from my case, telling me that they didn't get involved in individual human rights (despite their name), and that whilst I might feel that I had been the subject of prejudice, inequality and state-funded harassment, the Equality Act didn't apply to people like me.

Jeremy Hunt's office at the Department of Health and Social Care equally indulged in bland platitudes and also passed the matter back to the CQC.

Even the Patients' Association failed to respond to my requests for assistance.

HOWEVER, FOR SHEER HYPOCRISY, flaccid disinterest and dystopian doublespeak, the latest and last response from the Department of Health and Social Care surely takes pride of place.

With Matt Hancock having replaced Jeremy Hunt as Secretary of State for Health, Cat Smith (MP for Lancaster and Fleetwood) wrote again in late 2018, pleading for some kind of ministerial action over the ongoing punishment and detriment being suffered by myself and the family and the prospects of us not being reunited for another seven or eight years. Writing in response to Cat's plea for attention to my case, the letter was answered by Caroline Dinenege MP, and, at the time, a Minister of State for Care.

As an exercise in bland, meaningless platitudes and apathy, the response has few equals. But, as if to underline the utter hypocrisy of state and ministerial attitudes to whistleblowers, a quick search revealed the Right Honourable C. Dinenege to be MP for, of all places...Gosport!

Of course, it was Gosport where whistleblowers had been serially ignored or knocked back for over a decade, whilst hundreds of patients, allegedly, had their lives shortened by the activities of Dr Jane Barton.

Indulging, at the time of the Gosport revelations, in local media tub-thumping, shrill indignation and powerful damnation of those in power who had ignored or been indifferent to the pleas of local people, relatives and whistleblowers, Ms Dinenege clearly succeeded in projecting herself to the Gosport voters as a fearless defender of patients, NHS whistleblowers, responsible social disclosure, speaking up and safeguarding.

The perfect Minister and MP, surely, to at last show some true leadership and grit, put the rudderless regulators to shame, wade into, get involved and fearlessly champion the cause of a wronged NHS whistleblower and their struggle against corporate retaliation.

*So many people blew the whistle on this, so many families raised the alarm and there was just a failure to investigate by a number of different authorities...*thundered MP Caroline Dinenege on Sky News in June 2018.

We want our health and care system to be the safest and most compassionate in the world. This means encouraging patients to speak up with concerns, ensuring we act on them and learning from mistakes. I encourage anyone who has concerns over their care, or the care of loved ones, to share their experiences with the Care Quality Commission – so they can continue their vital work of protecting patients and improving the excellent care we see across the health service. Caroline Dinenege MP, Portsmouth, *The News* 2019.

These important measures should ensure staff can raise concerns knowing they are protected by the law and that their career in the NHS will not be damaged as a result of wanting to do the right thing.

We want to make the NHS the safest healthcare system in the world, so we must build a culture of openness and transparency among our staff.

For too long we have failed to protect those who are brave enough to speak out when others won't.... Caroline Dinenege MP, *Nursing Times* March 2018.

Yet, when powerful, moral, individual and ministerial leadership and courage was needed, as opposed to empty, sterile rhetoric, and with a truly perfect opportunity to come good on her authoritative oratory and criticisms of others, the response from the Right Honourable C Dinenege, MP and Minister of State for Care was, in my opinion, a masterclass in political insincerity, weakness, hypocrisy and doublespeak. Having postured for the benefit of local constituents, it was clear that, with her ministerial hat on, Ms Dinenege exactly epitomised the casual disinterest in whistleblower retaliation from those in power that had so recently defined the NHS disaster in her own electoral backyard.

Department of Health & Social Care

From Caroline Dinenage MP
Minister of State for Care

39 Victoria Street
London
SW1H 0EU

020 7210 4850

Your Ref: AS/ZA11263

PO-1163076

1 5 FEB 2019

Cat Smith MP
House of Commons
Westminster
London SW1A 0AA

Dear Cat,

Thank you for your further correspondence of 7 January to Matt Hancock on behalf of your constituent Mr Peter Duffy of   ,   , Lancaster LA1   about NHS whistleblowers.

I was sorry to read of Mr Duffy's continuing concerns. I hope he will understand that neither I nor the Secretary of State are currently able to accept his invitation to meet.

The *NHS Long-Term Plan*, published earlier this month, makes a commitment to making the NHS *a consistently great place to work*. This requires an open and transparent culture in which staff who speak up are supported in raising their concerns to help to make improvements for others.

As I wrote in November, the Department remains committed to ensuring appropriate, practical help and support is provided for staff who do raise concerns. It is important for both staff and patients that those concerns are taken seriously and properly investigated.

All healthcare professional regulators set standards and give advice for creating policies for raising and acting on concerns. This guidance expects organisations to ensure their policies make employees feel confident and are not penalised when raising concerns.

Following the legal duty requiring all prescribed bodies to publish an annual report on the whistleblowing disclosures made to them by workers, the healthcare professional regulators published a joint report in September, which can be found at www.gmc-uk.org by searching for 'whistleblowing report 2018'. It highlights the regulators' coordinated effort to manage raised concerns, ensure transparency in how disclosures are handled, highlight the action taken about these issues, and improve collaboration across the health sector.

220

Last year, we changed the law to protect whistle-blowers from discrimination when they seek re-employment in the NHS. We will continue to explore options to improve the support available to whistleblowers.

I hope this reply is helpful.

CAROLINE DINENAGE

Providing such an entirely and calculatedly unhelpful and disinterested response, stating that *the Department remains committed to ensuring appropriate, practical help and support for staff who raise concerns* whilst conspicuously offering precisely no departmental help or support whatsoever and going on to close with such a final sentence seemed, from my point of view, like little more than a thoroughly contemptuous political soldier's farewell and slap in the face.

Entirely predictably, neither Cat Smith nor myself ever heard from MP, Minister of State for Care and NHS whistleblower champion Ms Dinenege of Gosport ever again.

CHAPTER THREE

The Law

INTERNAL WHISTLEBLOWING ORGANISATIONAL POLICIES, promises and guardians, together with the regulators and Government ministers, as described above, appear to offer multiple safety nets where none actually exist. The law, on the other hand, definitely does offer a safety net. Where all else has failed, there certainly is a substantial legal structure beneath the falling whistleblower. However, whilst local, organisational, regulatory and ministerial promises and pledges of support might be likened to safety nets with all the robustness of cobwebs or moonbeams, the legal safety net might be best likened to one made of piano or cheese-wire. Not so much softly breaking and cushioning the whistleblower's fall, as much as slicing and dicing them on the way down.

The Public Interest Disclosure Act was introduced specifically to protect whistleblowers, so how has it become more of an instrument with which to damage and abuse them, above and beyond, of course, the corporate abuses and regulatory neglect that has already been inflicted upon them?

The answer, it seems to me, is not so much that it is poorly written (although it is certainly out of date), but that the due process of enforcing the law through the employment tribunal system seems to be prone to routine and cynical exploitation.

Most members of the public, especially *going solo* against a huge multi-billion pound state monopoly employer, end up being severely intimidated and outgunned by the process of litigation. Indeed, the process seems purpose designed to be intimidating. This is, arguably, with some good reason. Witnesses and participants in any process of law enforcement or litigation should be very fearful of breaching their legal responsibilities. Writing an honest sworn statement, giving accurate and truthful testimony under oath, not seeking to adversely influence other witnesses, dissuade them from appearing or tamper with their or your own evidence, declaring all evidence in your possession, whether it supports your case or not – these are all absolute legal obligations required of anyone or any organisation participating in a case of litigation. Furthermore, it is well established from multiple reviews and psychological profiling exercises that typical whistleblowers are hardworking, decent, straightforward, loyal employees and members of society.

Precisely the kind of qualities that might make a good, responsible and professional worker and member of the public. But perhaps not the kind of qualities best suited to defending yourself against the highly threatening and gladiatorial, attack-is-the-best-form-of-defence, stab-in-the-back, *smoke and mirrors*, all's-fair-in-love-war-and-litigation, wild-west shootout that has defined my experience of whistleblowing and contemporary employment law practice.

Few innocent whistleblowers will go into an employment tribunal perfectly prepared to indulge in evidential tampering and spoliation, erasure of entire witness accounts, intimidation, threats and withholding of statements. Yet, on the opposite side of the coin, the grizzled, battle-scarred and frequent flying veterans of NHS Trusts seem, in my opinion, not to be so inhibited. Whilst whistle-blowing law in the UK may be outdated and well overdue for an overhaul, any attempts to rewrite such laws to address current injustices are doomed to failure for as long as large organisations are allowed to continue to treat the procedures and mandatory standards of employment law and the judicial process with clear and present contempt.

Witnesses are an absolutely vital part of any court or tribunal process. As detailed in *Whistle in the Wind*, I'd expected to secure robust support and eyewitness evidence from a good six to twelve ex-colleagues from the urology department, booking a full two week hearing expressly for this purpose. Yet each and every one of my UHMBT witnesses dropped out after being very bluntly warned by the UHMBT medical hierarchy that the department might be *dissolved* in the event of the case concluding badly for the NHS.

The response of my legal team was one of shock. *They can't do that...!*

Except that the Trust did...and as a consequence of the fear that this statement generated, I failed to secure any witness evidence from a single one of my previously loyal UHMBT ex-colleagues. Perhaps unsurprisingly, bearing in mind some of the other tactics, the employment tribunal didn't seem particularly disturbed at this evidential and witness no-show and wastage of several days of tribunal time.

Of all my ex-colleagues, there was one in particular whose witness evidence I was most anxious to secure. Despite asking Colin Cutting in 2016 and at a very early stage to be a witness for me, he was robustly informed by UHMBT's management that he would only be allowed to appear as a witness for the NHS. Refusing to sign the witness statement drawn up for him, to his great credit he courageously insisted on writing his own. He was then, as a consequence, very bluntly informed by UHMBT that he'd not be appearing at all, and his witness statement and contained evidence would be withheld from the tribunal.

A recent NHS Freedom of Information request has now succeeded in securing a copy of Mr Cutting's withheld witness statement.

Just as might have been expected in *Nineteen Eighty-Four*, big brother couldn't resist erasing some of the evidence, and the alterations clearly cover a great deal more than just names. However, even without the evidence that has been blacked out, there is further clear proof and triangulation of my legal contention and central allegation that I had been the recipient of a sustained campaign of retaliation and retribution in response to my (and other people's) attempts to raise both personal and professional standards within the department.

Perhaps unsurprisingly, the NHS has refused point-blank to disclose the alternative witness statement – the one that was written out for Mr Cutting to sign by the NHS legal team, and which he refused to put his name to.

We can therefore only speculate upon the alternative facts that UHMBT's legal team expected Colin Cutting to present to the employment tribunal under oath.

Employment Tribunal Statement

The statement of ████████

I am currently one of the ████ ██████████ at MBHT. ███████████████████████
███████████████. One of the main reasons I applied for the ████████ job here was that I
had seen in ████ a ████████ who not only had excellent technical and clinical skills, but also
made caring for his patients his first priority.

██

We worked together for many years, and in ████ I saw someone who worked extremely
hard, who continued to have an exceptionally high standard of patient care and had the
most expertise, experience and surgical skill within the department.

Unfortunately, the department has had many ongoing difficulties. When concerns about
cases, clinical competence, honesty and professional attitudes have been raised, it has led
to those who raised the concerns coming under intense scrutiny. I have experienced this
recently myself. The stress and pressure of working in an environment where you know
that everything you do is being scrutinised, with colleagues looking to find fault, is immense.

████ has had to work with this stress for many years, following his raising concerns about a
colleague before I had even joined the department.

███████████████████████████████████████. This was only a small aspect of
my job (officially 2 out of 12 working sessions), as my main role was that of a ████████
primarily caring for patients. During my time, I tried to help develop the ████████
department and improve the ████████ service for our patients. I also had to manage any
departmental problems and concerns and I always tried to do this with openness,
transparency and fairness and to the best of my ability.

I was aware of the ongoing relational difficulties between ████ and other colleagues in the
department. The number of issues going on at one time was great, and given my limited
time, I did the best I could in trying to help deal with each incident and person as they arose.
███
███ to work with our
department to try and resolve some of our relational difficulties.

As a department we were really struggling to provide adequate cover for inpatients and
emergency admissions of ████████ patients at ████. The ██████████████████ would
cover all ████ inpatients and ████ emergencies at both ██ and ██ each weekday and
would drive between the sites to do the daily ward rounds. This was proving quite arduous
and stressful for the ██████████████ although it did ensure all ████ in-patients and
emergency admissions were seen at least every weekday and there was good continuity of
care.

At this time, ███ expressed to me how stressful he found it working at ███ due to the breakdown in relationship between him and some of the other ███ ███. He informed me that he felt threatened by them.

So in light of the on-call, Cross Bay work pressure and the stresses ███ felt working at ███ we as a department then discussed different job plan options to provide daily better care at ███ and reduce the travelling between sites for the ███████████████.

The option that we as a department, and ███ himself agreed to, was for ███ to cover all inpatients and emergencies at ███ on ██████████████████████, doing a morning and evening ward round each day and then doing set clinical activities such as operating or clinics for the rest of his time there. On ███████ he would continue to do his private practice in the morning and would do patient clinical administrative work in the afternoon (as his secretary was based at ███. On those days, ███ would be covered by our ██████████ ███████████.

██████████████████████████████job plan which as accurately as possible reflected the job plan above, including the time of travel from ███████ to ███. As this came out to significantly more than 12 PAs, which was deemed the maximum that the Trust would agree to, as part of a contract (although there are others in the Trust on more than a 12PA job plan), it was agreed that the additional working would be accounted for with 2 regular AAS (Additional Activity Sessions). I was lead to believe that regular Additional Activity Sessions could not be written into a contract but was also aware that many in the Trust, including other consultants in the ███████ department, were undertaking regular weekly AAS.

██████████████, I was involved in job planning but was not aware of my colleagues' salary scales or clinical excellence awards, which go to make up their overall salary. I always felt that, such specific financial matters were for our ████████████ and ███████ ██████████ to deal with. I know that there were emails back and forth about agreeing and signing things off, however this was now out of my remit.

I have tried to give a truthful overview of how I see the events unfolding.

My final summary is that our ███████ department has had immense difficulties, and the Trust have not resolved how we deal with colleagues that we have concerns about as to regards to their clinical competence, professional behaviour and attitudes. The backlash and ongoing stress of raising legitimate concerns and continuing to work within the department where there is an ongoing blame culture is immense. Even the most resilient eventually reach a breaking point.

███████ has been a valued colleague and a friend who I have great respect for. His reputation is that he is a hardworking, outstanding ███████ who has diligently served the population of Morecambe Bay.

MUCH OF THE TRIBUNAL ARGUMENT centred around whether I really had been the victim of a sustained anti-whistleblower campaign of abuse, harassment and disinformation with the aim of securing my dismissal or resignation, or whether I'd simply been dismissed, essentially *by accident*.... Mr Cutting's statement and sworn evidence would have been absolutely invaluable evidence, given by a neutral, impartial and extremely well-informed eyewitness.

Yet this vital evidence, testimony and witness statement was deliberately withheld from judicial scrutiny by the UHMBT legal team.

There can be no doubt that my case was very substantially weakened by the fact that I was ultimately unable to field any of my previous close UHMBT colleagues as witnesses. I have no doubt that, had they felt able to give a full and frank account without fear or favour, then they would have overwhelmingly and unanimously confirmed my case.

COLIN'S EVIDENCE WASN'T THE ONLY THING that *went missing* from UHMBT's legal requirement and obligation to declare all evidence for the purposes of justice and the tribunal.

Below is an innocent looking email string from the 7th July 2016; that fateful day when, amongst other things – with some £35,000 gone from my earnings and a threat, amongst other threats, to *'recoup'* further monies from my previous earnings, I finally felt compelled to throw in the towel on my NHS career and vocation with UHMBT.

This email string was presented as evidence to the employment tribunal as part of the legal bundle and to fulfil UHMBT's absolute legal requirement to disclose all evidence.

I have been legally advised to conceal the identity of the managers involved.

Reading from the top down, the email chain commences with my resignation email to Dr David Walker – then Medical Director.

Forwarded from David Walker to executive A at 11.47am, later the same day it is passed on to executive B at 12.45pm.

That evening, executive B *links* with both David Walker and manager C at 9.44pm, the email from executive B requesting that manager C assist Dr Walker with preparing a response, the string being forwarded on to manager D the following morning.

From: Duffy Peter (UHMB)
Sent: 07 July 2016 08:57
To: Walker David (UHMB)
Cc: ▇▇ ▇▇ (UHMB); ▇▇ ▇▇ (UHMB); ▇▇▇ ▇ (UHMB)
Subject: Resignation

Dear David

Please find attached my resignation letter from the Trust.

From: Walker David (UHMB)
Sent: 07 July 2016 11:47
To: Exec A ▇ (UHMB)
Subject: FW: Resignation

For info
David

From: Exec A ▇ (UHMB)
Sent: 07 July 2016 12:45
To: Exec B ▇ (UHMB)
Subject: FW: Resignation

From: Exec A (UHMB)
Sent: 07 July 2016 21:44
To: Man' C (UHMB); Walker David (UHMB)
Cc: (UHMB)
Subject: FW: Resignation

ψi

Can you please link with David to assist him in preparing a response to the attached.

Thanks

Regards,

University Hospitals of Morecambe Bay NHS Foundation Trust

From: Man' C (UHMB)
Sent: 08 July 2016 10:22
To: Man' D (UHMB)
Subject: FW: Resignation
Attachments: resignation letter.docx

fyi

All very reasonably in order and fitting nicely with executive B's sworn and signed statement to the tribunal, reproduced below.

The emphasis is mine.

> In turn I asked that ▮▮▮ liaise with Dr Walker in order to prepare a response to Mr Duffy's resignation [1658-1662]. That response was sent on 8 July 2016 by Dr Walker [1663-1664].
>
> But never received.
>
> Mr Duffy's employment ended on 26 September 2016 **and I was not involved in the interactions which took place between Mr Duffy's resignation and his employment ending**.

Executive B's statement to the employment tribunal (immediately above) together with the preceding email evidence all seems consistent with the overall UHMBT version of events formally put to the employment tribunal under oath.

Misunderstandings...a failure of anyone to definitively take charge, time drifting on with senior management distracted and perhaps a little too preoccupied with other things, the issue delegated to less senior managers, with other junior managers and accountants out of their depth, and a letter acknowledging my resignation that...*got lost in the post.* Overall, perhaps an NHS Trust not totally on the ball and in control of events. Maybe *a bit of a mix-up*...but most certainly not suggestive of a Trust that might have illegally forced a legitimate whistleblower out, reacted pretty much instantaneously to the resignation, and whose executive chain of command might, even within hours of that lone whistleblower finally crumpling and resigning under the pressure of illegal pay cuts and threats, have been working late and consulting with a firm of top, specialist lawyers. A legal team with a reputation for ruthlessness in their dealings with NHS whistleblowers, and with UHMBT following a clear, stated executive intent of planning for and heading off any potential litigation over the illegal dismissal of a whistleblower and the *inherent risks* in the situation.

Misunderstandings – another NHS favourite (not unlike *dysfunctional department*) and usually, in my experience, code for an act of bullying, abuse, harassment and suppression that didn't quite work out as expected. But from an employment tribunal scenario, not unreasonable, if very far-fetched to anyone familiar with the workings of NHS Trusts. *A genuine error.* Much regret and remorse over my resignation. UHMBT's executives slow to react but nothing planned, deliberate or anticipated. *A shame that it had to come to this.... The need for litigation much regretted*...etc.

Clearly, this was a version of events that the employment tribunal bought into, rejecting, after some deliberations, my own opinion that I'd been deliberately and knowingly forced out. That I'd made a nuisance of myself by speaking up to the regulators about an avoidable death, coronial contempt of court and facts that UHMBT desperately wanted to keep quiet. And that UHMBT's executive had actually been very well aware of my resignation right from the start and, far from being an *accident*, the Trust's executive had declined a number of opportunities to meet as part of what appeared to be a deliberate strategy, formulated with direct legal advice that was already being framed within hours of my forced resignation.

Very frustratingly, I'd known all along from contacts in the Trust that UHMBT had been galvanised into action right from the moment of my resignation. The organisation was, at the time, under significant pressure, both as a consequence of my external disclosures to the CQC and the backlash and retaliatory allegations of bullying and racism against myself from within the Trust. Additionally, and clearly aware of such counter allegations, both the BMA and BAPIO were looking over UHMBT's shoulders on behalf of my errant colleagues too, thereby putting even more pressure on senior executives. Of course, the UHMBT midwifery scandal and Kirkup Report, just months earlier, were still casting a long shadow across the Trust as well. With the Trust's handling of the issues in the urology department seeming to have already breached the public pledges made in the aftermath of the Kirkup Report, it was quietly but consistently suggested to me by several well connected sources that the executive UHMBT plan, worked out with high-level legal input, was to simply lie low, minimise contact with me, let me work out my resignation and hope that I disappeared quickly, silently and permanently from the scene.

In the meantime, UHMBT would quickly pull together a robust legal defence in the event that I didn't go quietly, and my illegal dismissal led to litigation.

Having submitted a number of Subject Access Requests in the run in to the tribunal, I was deeply disappointed that no written evidence turned up to corroborate the fact that UHMBT had been urgently taking detailed legal instructions and planning for whistle-blower litigation right from the day of my resignation. With any witnesses who might have confirmed this sequence of events having dropped out, and no declared disclosures backing up my *off the record* inside information, it was perhaps not surprising that the employment tribunal decided to go with UHMBT's *unfortunate accident and misunderstanding* version of events.

This, of course, tactically disconnected my illegal dismissal claim from my whistleblowing evidence and therefore dramatically pegged back any compensation, as documented in *Whistle in the Wind*.

Consultant A's hundreds of pages of allegations, detailed in the GMC allegations of Part I, chapter 5 have already demonstrated that hard evidence of multiple attempts to smear me as a bully and racist existed within multiple email accounts back in 2015 to 2018.

However, just as with the undisclosed evidence of the briefings and racism allegations against me in 2015, similar evidence also existed (but equally remained hidden), showing that, far from being a bit hands-off, casual and slow on the uptake; at least one UHMBT senior executive had been working very late into the evening, planning their response to my forced resignation and networking with Capsticks solicitors right from the very day that my resignation went in. That senior executive being, of course, exactly the same one who had made such categorical assurances, under oath, to the tribunal, that they'd had nothing to do with my case between my resignation going in and my final day of employment.

The following exchange was inadvertently revealed by UHMBT following a recent Subject Access Request, made well after the litigation was over.

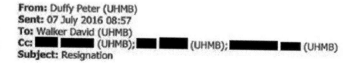

From: Duffy Peter (UHMB)
Sent: 07 July 2016 08:57
To: Walker David (UHMB)
Cc: ▮▮ ▮▮ (UHMB); ▮▮ ▮▮ (UHMB); ▮▮ ▮▮ (UHMB)
Subject: Resignation

Dear David

Please find attached my resignation letter from the Trust.

From: Walker David (UHMB)
Sent: 07 July 2016 11:47
To: Exec A ▮▮ (UHMB)
Subject: FW: Resignation

For info
David

From: ▓Exec A▓ (UHMB)
Sent: 07 July 2016 12:45
To: ▓Exec B▓ (UHMB)
Subject: FW: Resignation

From: ▓Exec B▓ UHMB)
Sent: 07 July 2016 21:46
To: ▓Exec A▓ (UHMB)
Subject: RE: Resignation

Thanks
I have asked   to support David with a response – I will suggest that she get a view of the draft from Capsticks before it goes out, I would like to try to minimise te potential risks inherent in the suggestion in the letter..

Regards,

University Hospitals of Morecambe Bay NHS Foundation Trust

From:	▓Exec A▓ (UHMB)
To:	▓Exec B▓ (UHMB)
Subject:	RE: Resignation
Date:	08 July 2016 08:11:47

OK – thanks.

So, in complete contrast with the previous declared email chain, and also in complete contradiction of executive B's sworn and signed affirmation that they were...*not involved in the interactions which took place between Mr Duffy's resignation and his employment ending* as per their sworn statement, this individual had, in reality, been working late into the evening on the very day I resigned. Not only helping to co-ordinate responses and actions with both Capsticks and a very senior executive within twelve hours of receipt my resignation, but also committing themselves to *minimising the potential risks,* a situation that could hardly be further removed from that individual's evidence under oath, offered to the Manchester Employment

Tribunal. And, of course, the exact opposite of the actions that would be expected of an organisation that, to its dismay, had just entirely accidentally triggered the forced resignation of its Doctor of the Year – a loyal and hardworking consultant and member of staff who had delivered fifteen years of committed front-line service.

There can be no doubt that, particularly as another, much more innocent sounding part of this email string was submitted, this crucially important evidence should have been formally declared to the employment tribunal. By selecting out and declaring only the innocent part and concealing a section that clearly demonstrated that UHMBT had been taking high-powered external legal advice within hours, and clearly discussing their near-instantaneous fears of the *potential risks inherent in the suggestions in the* (resignation) *letter*, it seems both clear and logical that UHMBT fundamentally misled the tribunal by withholding this evidence too. Additionally, executive B also would appear to have misled the panel by declaring under oath that they had had no involvement in my case between my resignation and my employment ending when, within hours of my resignation, this person was undoubtedly a key player, working late to co-ordinate UHMBT's response whilst factoring in expert legal advice and charting out the best way to minimise the potential legal consequences of the NHS's illegal dismissal of a whistleblower.

Clearly, UHMBT's management knew exactly what they were doing all along and, within hours of my forced resignation, were working late and taking external legal advice from an expert team of solicitors with a national reputation for dealing with potentially awkward whistleblower cases.

So, with written evidence withheld, all third-party UHMBT witnesses dropping out, false counter-allegations, my entire email account and all the evidence contained within being illegally destroyed, at least one sworn NHS witness statement that was fundamentally *economical with the actualité* over the reactions to my resignation, and another truthful written witness testimony deliberately withheld, by the time the first hearing arrived, there wasn't much left of the evidential process that hasn't already been adversely influenced and profoundly corrupted.

Except, of course, for the last bit of evidence.

The testimony still to come from the main witness themselves. The claimant and whistleblower.

10th April 2018

Dear Sirs

WITHOUT PREJUDICE SAVE AS TO COSTS

Mr Peter Duffy v University Hospitals Of Morecambe Bay NHS Foundation Trust Case Numbers: 2404382/2016 and 2406078/2016

We act for the Respondent, University Hospitals of Morecambe Bay NHS Foundation Trust, in this matter.

Costs Warning

For the reasons set out below, and having had the opportunity to review the documentation disclosed in this matter and your client's witness statements, we consider that your client's claims have no reasonable prospects of success and we invite your client to withdraw.

If your client does not withdraw his claim...we will make an application to the Tribunal for an order that your client pays some or all of our client's costs in defending the claim....

For the reasons set out above, we consider that your client's claims are misconceived, that none of your client's claims have any reasonable prospect of success and that their continued pursuit is unreasonable (and in some instances, vexatious).

We therefore invite your client to enter into a legally binding COT3 whereby your client withdraws his claim and each party bears its own costs and agrees not to make application for an order for costs against the other party. This will be on the standard COT3 terms that the deal done is without admission of liability, that neither party or its agents will make derogatory comments about the other, that the fact and terms will remain confidential....

This is the only offer that our client is willing to make.

For your information, my client's current legal fees expenditure on this matter is circa £65,000 plus VAT. It is estimated that this will be in the region of £90,000 plus VAT if this matter progresses to the 10-day final hearing.

We reserve the right to bring this letter to the attention of the Tribunal in support of any application for a costs order against your client if our client's offer is not accepted. We look forward to hearing from you.

Costs Threats

WHILST LITIGATION IS A CONFRONTATIONAL and bruising process, there can surely be no excuse for such aggressive and intimidating language, especially when the legal firm involved had already mistakenly submitted documentation to the tribunal, clearly but accidentally conceding that their client (UHMBT) most certainly <u>had</u> illegally withheld monies from my earnings (see *Whistle in the Wind*, page 178). Far from my case being unreasonable, vexatious and having no reasonable prospect of success, in actual fact, the NHS knew full well that I had a *prima-facie*, cut and dried case of illegal pay deduction and that, in fact, if complete truth had been honestly told to the tribunal, it was the NHS that was trying to defend the utterly indefensible.

Nevertheless, it was clear at this point in the litigation that UHMBT and their legal team were intent on either bullying and harassing me into backing down, or alternatively abusing the legal process sufficiently (albeit within the parameters of what is legally acceptable) to attempt to inflict maximum revenge financial damage upon my family.

In the end, the *costs warning,* whilst not succeeding in intimidating me into silence, persuading me to drop the case and agree to a gag, did at least, from UHMBT's point of view have the desirable effect of compelling me to hastily reduce and rewrite my case, materially weakening it in order to try and guard against such a threat.

Astonishingly, this action in reducing my case, as a direct consequence of the original UHMBT threat of costs, then resulted in yet another attempt to claim costs, with the Trust later claiming that I had wasted its time by reducing my case, and bizarrely then trying to claim costs from me in compensation for the direct consequences of its original groundless costs threat! Such is the surreal, brutal and Kafkaesque world of anti-whistleblower litigation and legal tactics. Yet, whilst the manoeuvres and legal logic may be complex, from the whistleblower's point of view, it is plain and simple bullying and corruption of the legal process. A vast monopolistic organisation bolstered with unlimited taxpayer's funds, blatantly threatening, harassing and intimidating a solitary individual and their family with ruinous costs, whilst quietly hiding facts, witnesses and evidence that would fatally undermine its own case.

Precisely the kind of legal abuse that employment tribunals were set up to avoid.

It is also worth making the point that, as mentioned above, by this point in the litigation, my UHMBT email account and all the thousands of emails and evidence contained within it had been illegally erased. In this context, the Civil Procedure Rules of the Courts of England and Wales are particularly relevant in relation to evidential preservation, as quoted more fully earlier in Part I, chapter 14.

Failure to preserve all potentially disclosable documents when litigation is contemplated may also give rise to very serious sanctions, including costs sanctions, the striking out of a party's particulars of claim or defence...and/or the drawing of adverse inferences as to the contents of those documents.

So, here was UHMBT and their legal team authorising and threatening life changing costs, telling me that in essence I had no case and attempting to bully me into dropping my action. Yet all the time they were quietly holding back the fact that, as well as concealing evidence, a huge act of illegal evidential destruction had gone on at the heart of the case that would, had this been revealed to the tribunal, have potentially resulted in the collapse of their case, a default verdict against them and even the awarding of costs in the opposite direction.

When it comes to acts of corporate bullying, hypocrisy, illegality, abuses of process and corruption, it remains my opinion that this case fundamentally debases judicial standards and sets a whole new UK legal low.

The courts themselves have made clear that the standard of honesty required for solicitors and legal professionals is so high as to ensure that 'every member, of whatever standing, may be trusted to the ends of the earth' (Bolton v Law Society 1993).

The most astonishing inditement of the employment tribunal process is the realisation that, in the process of my illegal dismissal and subsequent litigation, UHMBT, their medical hierarchy, executives and legal team managed to inflict upon me and my family every single one of the established whistleblower punishments and detriments listed by the Westminster *All-Party Parliamentary Group* (APPG) on whistleblowing (see next chapter). Not only this, but the penalties, punishments and detriments happened in almost the perfect chronological order, as predicted by the APPG too.

This anti-whistleblower cycle of abuse is fully detailed in the following postscript and need not be addressed in detail here. But, of course, this observation leads to the inevitable and pivotal question that dwarfs all the other procedural issues that corrupted the entirety of the legal and employment tribunal process.

The tribunal accepted unanimously that I had been illegally and unfairly dismissed. Additionally, in spite of all the attempts at evidential concealment and witness intimidation, there remained clear and overwhelm-

ing evidence that, despite some fifteen years of straightforward, successful, productive, largely happy and uncontroversial employment, once I'd blown the whistle to the CQC, UHMBT, their executives, senior medics and legal team managed to inflict each and every single one of all of the well-recognised whistleblower detriments listed by the APPG upon myself and my family, somehow concentrating them all into the horribly abusive, bullying and miserable last 18 months of my NHS employment, illegal dismissal and the subsequent legal bloodbath.

So how on earth did the tribunal still manage to come to the callow, naïve and unworldly-wise conclusion that my illegal dismissal, within months of speaking out, was nevertheless simply a series of accidents? That all the myriad of well established, validated and documented whistleblower abuses that littered the wake of my last few months of NHS employment were simply coincidences, misunderstandings, happenstance and bad luck, rather than UHMBT following an extremely well established, well-beaten and choreographed pathway of whistleblower retaliation and abuse?

A cycle of institutional, state sponsored abuse and retaliation that is so well established that, without being at all aware of my case, the Westminster All-Party Parliamentary Group on whistleblowing were able to accurately predict and map out every single step of the corporate retaliation against myself and my family over the 18 month long death-throes of my surgical vocation in the NHS.

I'M WALKING ACROSS A NARROW BRIDGE. All around me there is noise and bustle. The smell of burnt diesel and soot fills my lungs and I look down on to the platform and railway lines through the grimy Victorian iron lattice at the side of the passenger footbridge.

A train screeches to a halt below me, and the jarring note of the PA system cuts through the air, echoingly announcing a new arrival. People push past, heads down and oblivious to anyone else.

And suddenly I'm aware of a family walking below me, heading towards and then underneath the footbridge that I'm standing on. With a sudden jolt and shock, I realise that I'm looking down at three little boys and a couple. There's Edward, holding his mother's hand and looking up intently into her face. Robert and William are clutching soft toys and gazing around in wonder at the trains and commotion. Fiona looks younger, wearing a dress that I haven't seen in at least fifteen years. And there's me...pushing the double buggy. More upright, fewer wrinkles and with a head of hair that I haven't seen in the mirror for well over a decade.

The family continue to walk towards me. Looking down, I can see every detail of their faces as I peer longingly through the ironwork of the bridge. There's a tenderness, affection and closeness about this small group that draws me irresistibly in, as though the family are highlighted; framed in colour and warmth, and everything else is painted in cold shades of grey. I so much want to get nearer, and share that quiet familiarity and intimacy, but I know I shouldn't. As though I'm aware of my own contagion and toxicity, and the danger that I pose to this intimate family group, I instinctively sense that I mustn't approach too near to them.

Passing beneath me, the family disappear behind the wrought iron guardrail and are gone.

And then I'm running frantically, weaving between groups of people, casting left and right. They won't have gone far, but I can't see them anywhere. Down the steel tipped stairs three at a time, sprinting down a platform edge. A train rushes past, just inches away and someone shouts at me, but I don't care. I'm focussed only on getting another glimpse of that family and sensing again that love; that easy, trusting bond, warmth and familiarity.

But with a lurch in my stomach and terrible sense of sadness and loss, I see the doors close on the other side of the platform. Accompanied by the strident revving of diesel engines, the carriages gradually begin to move

241

away from me and, with their backs to me, the family – my family; oblivious to my presence, are drawn slowly, agonisingly away and out of sight.

With an overwhelming, exquisitely sharp and painful sense of loss, like a knife through the ribs and to the heart, I realise that they are gone, and I'm left alone in a cold, grey, hostile world of chaos, loneliness, noise and strangers.

———————

THE EARLY MORNING LIGHT is seeping in around the blind. The seagulls are crying in the distance and I hear the clock tower in Peel striking six. It'll soon be time to wake from a slumber in which I never feel fully relaxed and asleep, and go to a job where I never really feel fully alive and awake. But there's perhaps another 45 minutes. Huddling back under the warm duvet, maybe, I think to myself, I can rekindle that dream; relieve again those moments of a life now forever lost, hide again under the covers and be carried away. Away back to a happier time and a place that, in this vicious, jagged, hurt-filled and discordant new existence, dominated by and overflowing with hate, cruelty and prejudice, I know, in cold reality, to have been brutally torn away from my grasp and to be gone...for good and forever.

POSTCRIPT

Cover-up and Carry-on

THE CYCLE OF WHISTLEBLOWER ABUSE[13]

1. *Reporting: The whistleblower decides to make a disclosure, often after longstanding concerns and discussions with colleagues, managers and family members;*

2. *Isolation: The organisation starts distancing itself from the whistleblower in several ways, such as by excluding them from the processes following the reporting, by isolating them and/or by turning staff against them. This can be accompanied by intimidation or harassment by the organisation.*

3. *Scrutiny: The organisation initiates a close scrutiny of the whistleblower and their work performance to discredit them. A previous high performer can suddenly become an underperformer, and whistleblowers can be set up to fail with impossible workloads or deadlines. Sometimes, whistleblowers are explicitly blamed for blowing the whistle.*

4. *Counter-accusations: The organisation moves informal accusations against the whistleblower, as part of a strategy as 'character assassination'...or to induce them to change their statements;*

5. *Disciplinary action: In many cases accusations are formally brought by the organisation against whistleblower through disciplinary proceedings which can culminate in sanctions. This not only discredits the whistleblower, but can be used by the organisation*

---

[13] https://www.appgwhistleblowing.co.uk/.

against them in court proceedings, especially before employment tribunals;

6. *Demotion/Pay reduction: Several negative consequences might follow or accompany the attempts to undermine or intimidate the whistleblower, including demotion from a role or a location and reduction in salary or other benefits;*

7. *Dismissal/Forced resignation: The most serious formal way to retaliate against employee is dismissal or forced resignation;*

8. *Non-Disclosure Agreement (NDA): The organisation forces the whistleblower to sign a non-disclosure agreement preventing them from spreading their disclosure any further;*

9. *Allegations ignored/case closed: Discrediting, silencing or removing the whistleblower allows the organisation to ignore or dismiss the allegations made in their disclosure.*

AS WE APPROACH the second birthday of *Whistle in the Wind*, has anything been learned? Or, as a society, are we still stuck in the same Kafkaesque rut of risk-taking, whistleblower abuse, counter-allegations, fear, cover-up, regulatory blindness and the wilful manipulation of evidence?

There seems no doubt about the answer.

THE PREDICTABLE AND CHOREOGRAPHED abuse of whistleblowers, both in the public and private sectors is a well established phenomenon. Studied in a number of countries, it is remarkable how similar and ingrained the patterns of ill-treatment are, regardless of nationality, culture, religion and geography.

Various authors and authorities have pointed out the corrupt, repeating and predictable cycle of abuse that awaits the vulnerable whistleblower. One of the better researched and substantiated articles was published by the UK's All-Party Parliamentary Group on whistleblowing, whose *cycle of abuse* is detailed above and referred to in the last chapter.

For those familiar with *Whistle in the Wind*, it is clear that, between them, the NHS, the regulators and the law inflicted every single one of these anti-whistleblower sanctions upon myself and my family.

Only two of these whistleblower detriments failed to stick. In 2016, an attempt to commence a disciplinary process failed, and, of course, an attempt was made to impose a non-disclosure order or gag (a COT3 in my case) as a part of the *costs warning* in 2018.

Careful scrutiny of this cycle of abuse is not a dry, academic exercise. As NHS disaster after disaster has shown, repeated nationwide failures of candour and safeguarding within this monopoly employer have inflicted so much suffering and avoidable death. Nevertheless, judging from my recent experiences, we are no further towards finding a solution that might genuinely promote a culture of learning and safety, whilst protecting those tasked with the responsibility for safeguarding the public from the suffocating weight of organisational secrecy, spin, manipulation and institutional retaliation.

As alluded to in the prologue, such cultures of covert cover-up are by no means confined to the NHS, or to just the state sector. Internationally, the Boeing 737 Max disasters inevitably lead to the question of just how many employees and engineers knew that the company was installing hardware and software to compensate for an ageing design that might, with one malfunction, wrest control from the pilots and plunge the plane into an uncontrollable dive? Why didn't more people come forward and speak out, particularly after the first crash? And for those courageous few who did, why were they not listened to?

Closer to home, how many people in the construction industry knew that high-rise housing blocks were being sheathed in insulating material that could potentially turn the whole building into a blazing inferno within minutes? Yet it took the wholly unnecessary loss of many dozens of lives, lives taken in unimaginable pain and terror – some of them babies and young children, to bring such clear and ever-present dangers to light.

WHISTLE IN THE WIND teased out a number of failings. These have been further elaborated and detailed in *Smoke and Mirrors* and several wholly new punishments, retaliations and detriments have made it into the discourse. Broken corporate promises and examples of NHS *doublespeak*. Violations of candour and the law at every conceivable level together with an ongoing and obsessional devotion to spin and cover-up, even when it involves the use of clearly fabricated and misleading evidence. Regulatory blindness, weakness, laziness and wilful disinterest. And, of course, a legal system which appears, at least according to my own experiences, to openly tolerate, and thereby nurture and encourage the deliberate spoliation of evidence, witness intimidation and, of course, the terrifying threat of *costs*.

But, over and above these multitudinous state and organisational failings, in themselves bewildering in their variety and endless permutations, can we find a single factor that can be identified? A common, universal shortcoming and unifying characteristic behind the domino effect of sequential flaws and missed opportunities, often going back many years? A behavioural weakness that condemns our society to suffering more avoidable disasters and, equally, condemns potential whistleblowers to the ongoing reality of lies, bullying, fabrications, retaliation and *smoke and mirrors*? And perhaps, looking at the inverse of this failing, is it possible to define characteristics that, bestowed upon our institutions in greater quantity, might help us to avoid yet more avoidable deaths, harm and near misses in the future?

FIVE YEARS OF EXILE; empty, blank and meaningless weekends, dark, solitary evenings and long, lonely journeys back to a home that, increasingly, feels like somewhere I used to live in a previous life; all of these have given me plenty of time to review and refine my opinions on the events of the last decade. And, with two more years having passed since the publication of *Whistle in the Wind*, much of it spent in total isolation from my family and friends, there has been ample opportunity to hone and develop the limited views that I expressed in 2019.

Digging ever deeper into the details of my last decade of experience of the NHS is a revealing, sordid and deeply depressing exercise, as more and more acts of hypocrisy, weakness, dishonesty, bullying, illegality, harassment, cover-up and corruption come to light.

But what is the defining characteristic if we go in the opposite direction? Instead of focussing on the fine detail, what do we see, writ large, by instead stepping back and taking a wider viewpoint from the perspective of both my experiences and that of others? The forest of failures over whistleblowing, professional standards and safeguarding, rather than the individual leaves and branches?

The answer, of course, underpinning this entire, decade long catalogue of failure from senior medics, executives, organisations, regulators, senior politicians and the law, weaving these all together into an almost seamless continuum is, time and time again, poor quality, short-sighted, ineffectual and amoral leadership.

Looking back to Part III, chapter 1, the common factor binding together the disastrous decisions that characterised the management of the urology department over many years was, in the end, weak, vacillatory senior NHS leadership. A failure to robustly confront risk-taking and bad behaviour, a failure to support those who were trying to raise standards, and a collective corporate failing of courage in the face of poor patient outcomes, behavioural issues, covert, defamatory briefings and retaliation.

As detailed in Part III, chapter 2, the regulators, guardians, commissioners and Department of Health and Social Care showed a similar and singular lack of moral courage and leadership too. Just as with UHMBT, there was no shortage of official rhetoric and promises, no lack of exhortations and incentives to staff to speak up and safeguard. Just a woeful and wilful lack of mindful, moral mettle and leadership and a clear desire that someone else; or some other organisation step in, do the heavy lifting and display the requisite courage and moral governance.

Of course, no one did, with my case being passed around amongst the regulators, government departments and authorities like a game of pass the parcel, except with everyone behaving as though the parcel contained a particularly repulsive forfeit.

And looking at Part III, chapter 3, the law and the tribunal process, can we tease out any examples of mindful and courageous leadership from the events of 2017 and 2018, or was this too, a moral, lawless wasteland? Paras Gorasia and Chris Thompson, my employment tribunal lawyers, were clear exceptions to the rule. I was lucky to be advised by them, and they were prescient in warning me that, right from the start, I ought to brace myself for some seriously prejudiced and abusive behaviour. But in the end, never; not even in my worst nightmares could I have anticipated the moral and legal vacuum and whirlwind of disingenuity, disinformation and dishonesty that I'd get sucked into.

In this context of legal failings and poor leadership, it is worth examining the relationship between the written law, and the way in which that written law is assessed, interpreted and enforced. In the UK, the Public Interest Disclosure Act (PIDA) forms the legal bedrock upon which employment and whistleblowing cases are built.

Coming in for much criticism, it is nevertheless worth pointing out that the PIDA was not, in itself, a bad attempt at providing support and legal backup for wronged whistleblowers. Properly interpreted through a rigidly policed, evenly balanced and truly impartial legal process, it should have been a very valuable addition to whistleblower protections.

What has led to this well intentioned act being widely regarded as effete and obsolete?

The answer, of course is, once more, poor, amoral leadership.

Underpinning any judicial process is the ubiquitous, legal and mandatory requirement of respect for truth, honesty and full, candid disclosure of all evidence by the legal teams on both sides, whether it be written, electronic or eyewitness. Those legal teams, according to the legal profession's own definitions, being of sufficient integrity to be *trusted to the ends of the earth.* And with the NHS itself using taxpayer's funds that had been earmarked for healthcare purposes to underwrite and direct its legal case against me, the high moral requirements of the legal process should have been further buttressed by the NHS Constitution and the Nolan principles; a non-negotiable code of conduct to which all public sector organisations must adhere.

Integrity, selflessness, objectivity, leadership, accountability, openness, honesty.

Yet, in the corrupt legal bloodbath that followed, each and every one of these qualities was entirely absent.

With the comprehensive debasing of the legal and litigation process listed in Part III, chapter 3, it is difficult to see how the tribunal processes of 2018 could have possibly moved further away from the ethics and practice of the law, the Nolan principles and the NHS Constitution.

And herein lies another major legal flaw in this process. The Public Interest Disclosure Act may be far from perfect, but even the most tightly written laws in the world would have failed in the face of such a miserable collapse in the moral and ethical standards that should underpin the process of litigation. What characteristic underlies this failure? Once again, poor, craven leadership; a complete absence of powerful moral authority from those driving the case and overseeing the legal process against me, and a weak and corrupt drive to win at all costs. So very far away from proper, strong and ethical leadership, which could and should, after a careful study of the case, have produced a dignified admission of liability and sincere regret, an unshakeable intent to do as much as was necessary to put things right, and a powerful and enduring commitment to learn and do better next time.

———————

POOR, TIMOROUS AND OFTEN ABSENT LEADERSHIP runs through the ten year history of these events like the words embedded in a decade long stick of Blackpool rock. No matter which part is sliced or how you view the cut end, the characteristic is always there. Scrutinising the accounts of other public and private sector whistleblowers and comparing with my own story, the lack of clear, safety orientated, moral and courageous custodianship and executive direction is an almost constant factor, there for all to see, with a persistent and weak reversion to cover-up, bullying, intimidation, tolerance of low standards, suppression of bad news and tactical blindness. Not only does this leave the vulnerable at risk, but ultimately, such lack of action simply emboldens those who feel that they can get away with lax, tainted standards and risk-taking. A downward spiral ensues, with reversion to *Smoke and Mirrors* whenever a difficult or embarrassing problem presents itself, a repetitive tendency to take the easy way out and an arrogance that, through manipulation, spin, harassment, the wearing down of individuals or just sheer financial and legal might, big monopolistic organisations like NHS Trusts will always be able to bluster, bludgeon, manipulate and muscle their way out of any embarrassing lapses of standards.

BUT IT'S EASY TO CRITICISE, isn't it? Especially with hindsight.

If we can identify failed or inadequate leadership, what might characterise the opposite? What features might we look for in individuals who could provide the kind of moral, civil, mindful, courageous public sector leadership that might finally put an end to this national, and indeed global cycle and scandal of corporate failings, whistleblower retaliation and state cover-up and carry-on?

We instinctively think of powerful national figures when we consider leadership. Characters forged out of war and national struggles. In the context of leadership of a safer, fairer, more social and civil society, we are, perhaps, better looking away from historical wartime leaders for that ethereal, gentler quality of true civil and social leadership. Gandhi, Luther King and Mandela perhaps, rather than Churchill, Napoleon or Thatcher. What qualities transform otherwise ordinary people into convincing, charismatic and compassionate civil, moral leaders, and what particular characteristics might mark out the next generation of NHS trailblazers, influencers, clinical and corporate leaders, who could break with past failures, take a less spineless position on risk-taking and cover-ups and be genuine and robust supporters of candour, high standards and public safeguarding?

The characteristics that most define such mindful, altruistic leadership are those of courage and compassion, the two melding together to forge a focussed, unwavering, lifelong, selfless commitment to bettering the lives and circumstances of others. But there can be no courage or bravery without risk. Each truly great and celebrated social and civil leader has been defined by their steadfast, energetic and selfless determination to lead and drive our societal evolution ever forward, whatever the personal risks and obstacles.

This is the kind of civil leadership that our culture needs to foster and nurture for all of our futures, and nowhere more than in our public services, where billions of pounds-worth of hard-earned taxpayer's money is consumed, putatively to benefit us all, but all too often disproportionally benefiting a select few. Not a single one of the world's truly great compassionate and inspiring societal leaders ever chose their roles for lavish wealth, the subjugation of others, prestige, job security, titles, a plush company car and a bottomless pension pot. And whilst most public services cannot realistically hope for a 21st century Gandhi, Mandela or Luther King at the helm, it surely shouldn't be difficult to aspire to having our state institutions led by individuals who at least seek to approach the qualities of these truly great and universally respected leaders.

But who directs our public sector and corporate leaders? Who polices and holds to account the non-executives and the regulators; those who, in turn, are supposed to continually assess, evaluate and restrain our big organisations and companies? Ultimately, it falls to our elected national politicians and ministers to regulate, temper, interpret and enforce the democratic and public safety principles that underpin our society.

When huge, monolithic state structures begin to crack and fail, when public service values are ignored and the internal checks and balances within such organisations are quietly switched off or disabled, when moral values like those expounded in Nolan's principles are flouted, insulted and roundly ignored, and when our national care and quality regulators prove to be asleep on the job, it falls to ministers and senior, national level politicians to lead and to show incisive courage and commitment. To steer our state structures and regulators away from the dangerous, dark and dingy depths of our current corporate and state obsessions with control, spin, suppression of bad news or perceived criticism, and into the sunlit uplands of candour, learning, high standards, safeguarding, state and corporate openness and integrity. Yet, once again, as exemplified by the events of Part III, chapter 2, my own experiences are of our national structures left rudderless; cast adrift, without any decisive, clear moral, principled senior political and ministerial guidance and helmsmanship.

Our privileged governmental principals, holding down their dominant and controlling posts in Westminster and Whitehall should not shirk their obligations in this regard – their responsibilities to those of us who work hard for our society and fulfil our part of societal moral obligations. Nowhere in our culture is there a greater need for courageous, compassionate and moral leadership than in our political leaders and ministers. And yet, despite the power, privilege and prerogatives of such societal elevation; nowhere, over the last five years and in my own experiences, has there been a greater vacuum of courageous, civic, ethical decision making and political guidance than at the very apex of our current, contemporary democratic pyramid.

And without the clear, defining moral helmsmanship from national politicians and ministers that our precious and fragile democracy requires and deserves; without determined, spirited civil leadership, a self-effacing drive to embed and enforce societal values of mutual respect, care, honesty, consideration and candour, we and those who follow us are simply damned to endlessly reprise our role as the victims of this same endless, costly, utterly corrupt and entirely avoidable cycle of corporate and governmental *smoke and mirrors.*

Epilogue

OUR DAILY LIVES ARE strewn by potential obstacles and harms. All around us we see and hear of people killed, injured, suffering or dying prematurely, and life itself is, of course, an epidemic of injustices. Who can, for example, coldly rationalise or dismiss the cot death that I witnessed as a callow young medical student, referred to in *Whistle in the Wind?*

I still recall it as though it was yesterday.

The horrific snuffing out of a tiny, vulnerable, beautiful, priceless and innocent young life; a life barely started – and, of course, the enduring pain still-to-come for the young and bereaved mother under such terrible circumstances.

Suffering, and the ever-present risk of death are both ubiquitous and are our constant companions through life. So much of this risk is accidental or unavoidable; inexplicable except possibly, to some higher deity, power or intelligence with access to a superior logic and insight that, despite our best efforts, we are not privileged to share.

However, there is also eminently avoidable suffering, danger and death which can, by its very definition, be prevented. Whilst such events may comprise only a small proportion of the daily hazards that we all face, there can be no possible excuse in any moral, well-led society for continuing to tolerate and cover-up the cynical, selfish and morally repugnant taking of avoidable risks with the lives and health of our fellow human beings.

And in this context it is, perhaps, one of the greatest indictments of our current culture that so very little effort is put into supporting and protecting the lives, sanity, careers and health of those who step out from the safety of the corporate line-up in order to discharge their moral, social and societal duties and attempt to intervene and safeguard the lives and health of others. Instead, state and private companies across the world devote vast amounts of time, energy, money and manpower to seeking out and silencing those who might break ranks and threaten those carefully cultured and manicured organisational reputations and balance sheets.

As a society, we can never eliminate risk, ill-health or premature death, but we absolutely owe it to our fellow citizens to do everything within our power to minimise these hazards. There is nothing that can be done now for the victims of avoidable medical and non-medical disasters – those who have paid with their health or with their lives, except, of course, to unequivocally commit to learn, improve and do better. And in the process, perhaps, adapt to listen constructively to those who might have safety-critical insights that are lacking at higher levels in the state or the organisation. As a society and a civilisation, we need to support, listen to and empower such individuals, rather than relapsing into the historical, feudal, corrupt and feral reflex of vilification, retaliation, harassment, vicious and vindictive bullying and illegal acts of detriment, cruelty, punishment and evidential manipulation.

AS WITH *Whistle in the Wind*, I very much hope that this book will stimulate people to both thought and action, and I am deeply grateful to each and every reader for considering my account. Please share this manuscript, publicise it via your social media connections; discuss with friends and family, and involve your local MP.

It is, as above, too late to save those who have already suffered, had their lives unnecessarily shortened, or died needlessly. Too late, too, to save the careers of those who have spoken out and paid the ultimate vocational price for their candour and integrity. But we can all play a role in fostering a new working environment where these injustices are consigned to history. It is only when our society itself appreciates and demands the selection, support and promotion of kindness, candour, honesty, learning and true leadership in the next generation of civic and national leaders, standard-bearers and influencers, ensuring that they possess the requisite empathy, moral courage and suitability to spearhead our great caring institutions, holding them to account and ensuring a durable commitment to safety and truthfulness that we can properly embed within our culture a ubiquitous philosophy of openness, quality, care and compassion, for ourselves, our loved ones, and those who will come after us.

Peter Duffy.
Peel,
Isle of Man.

28th May 2021.

ADDENDUM

Déjà Vu

THERE WASN'T ANY WARNING, simply a GMC email out of the blue, late on Wednesday afternoon, the 2nd June.

Summer 2021. The distinctly non-cathartic and disturbing construction of *Smoke and Mirrors* is nearly complete but unpublished, and, in stark contrast to the situation at the beginning of Part I chapter 1, the traumas and horrors of the NHS's, Manchester Employment Tribunal's and Niche Consulting's treatment of me are all too alive and well – back with a daily and nightly vengeance, in my consciousness, my subconsciousness, my daily work and in my disturbed sleep.

From: ▮▮▮▮ *(0161 923 6485)* <▮▮▮▮▮▮▮>
Date: Wed, 2 Jun 2021 at 17:03
Subject: Email from the General Medical Council

Dear Mr Duffy.

I am writing to let you know that we have received some information from ▮▮▮▮▮▮▮ *and NICHE which we need to investigate. I enclose a copy of the documents.*

Please also find attached a letter which provides more information about the investigation, what you need to do next and how to get support.

Please do not hesitate to contact me should you have any questions about the matters or wish to discuss anything in relation to the investigation.

Kind Regards

▮▮▮▮

Investigation Officer
General Medical Council
3 Hardman Street, Manchester M3 3AW

———————————

OH NO…NO…NO…NO…. *Please no…. For Heaven's sake! Surely not this again?? How many more times?*

I'm standing in the garden of our lovely family home in Lancaster.

It's summer. The trees are all in leaf, the sun strong; the lawns neatly mown and the beds are a mass of flowers and buzzing with insects. The birds are singing, with swallows twittering, wheeling and darting over my head. Fiona and the boys are relaxing in the house, perhaps looking forward to one of Fiona's exceptional roast lunches, and the kittens are peacefully asleep in their basket. Everything is as it should be....

But there's some cloud in the distance.

It grows denser, even as I watch. Grey cumulus mutates into an ugly, unhealthy and repulsive looking dark grey and orange monstrosity. The cloud begins to boil and, from its root, writhing, evil-looking tentacles reach down to the ground. Twisting and gyrating like ghoulish, tortured serpents, I see debris rising from where the tentacles reach the earth, distant house roofs being torn down and flung in the air, trees ripped up, terrified birds sucked helplessly into the vortex....

I'm rooted to the spot as the nearest tornado twists and writhes towards me. A bright flash lights up the darkened, boiling sky as the vortex slices through and shorts out power cables. Sparks fly up into the whirling, seething maelstrom and, with mounting panic, I see the squirming, flaming column of smoke and fire approaching the back of our lovely house....

I'm trying to shout out to the family, but my weak pleadings are lost in the roar of the storm.

The windows disintegrate, sucked inwards in a cloud of razor shards of lethal glass. Our beautiful family home implodes around the foot of the tornado; one second, it, and the family are there, and the next second....

My feet thud to the floor of the flat and I'm standing upright, pouring sweat, heart hammering with *the towering fiery maelstrom soaring and writhing right over my head....*

But no, it's fading...the storm-winds blowing in my face and crackle of electricity and fire in my ears dissipates, and I'm left, wringing wet, head down, trembling and panting for breath and with just the distant plaintive seagull cries and the dark, lonely silence of the flat.

1.30am.

Peel,
Isle of Man.

And somehow, I've got to be fit to operate in the morning.

When is this going to end?

TIMELINE

A recap of events leading up to the publication of Whistle in the Wind

THOSE READERS WHO HAVE only recently finished *Whistle in the Wind* or who are intimately acquainted with the story can ignore this summary. However, for those not immediately familiar with the chronology, a quick refresh of events is necessary to put the chapters of Part I into the correct context.

Many of the events subsequent to the employment tribunal tend to diverge and lead the reader in all sorts of confusing and contradictory directions, especially for those following the story who are not familiar with the medical profession, General Medical Council, NHS and other regulatory bodies.

This should not be unexpected. One of the regular tactics employed against those who speak up is the deployment of counter allegations, along with confusing and contradictory statements, half-baked enquiries, 'new' and confusing evidence, and so on. The clear intent, in my opinion, is to bog down patients, relatives, regulators and interested member of the public to such an extent that they give up, considering that they will never be able to make sense of so many contradictions and complications.

Bear with me, and hopefully this chapter will help the interested reader to navigate the minefield of misinformation, some of it undoubtedly deliberate, that lies ahead.

Rather than giving a simple timeline of dates and events, this chapter will concentrate on walking the reader forwards through the major, pivotal events from around 2012 onwards, and then, from the point of publication of *Whistle in the Wind*, take the story still further forward as it splits and diverges into multiple different fragments, each of which will hopefully be brought back together to fully crystallise the whole story in the separate chapters of Part I.

———————

2000 to 2010. UHMBT appoints and employs me as consultant urological surgeon. Despite some early issues over clinical standards in the department, the job goes well and, after two decades of training in London and SE England, I feel that my vocation is well on the way to being fulfilled.

2012. After one of my consultant colleagues returns from retraining, Mrs Irene Erhart dies from poorly treated uro-sepsis at Furness General Hospital. The coroner concludes that her care was far from optimal.

2013. Further concerns begin to be raised within the UHMBT department of urological surgery about standards, particularly in reference to the attention given to emergency and acutely ill urology patients.

2014. A colleague is suspended for the second time after, amongst other things, mistakenly listing a patient with cancer to have the wrong kidney removed.

Late 2014. A number of incidents happen, including a patient being discovered who is due to be sent home without intervention and with a large and untreated bladder cancer, obstructed kidneys and blood tests suggesting possible sepsis. Another *Clinical Incident* form is submitted.

Very late 2014. A meeting is called with UHMBT management where, unknown to myself, allegations of racism are made against me by the individuals who I have expressed concerns about. At least one external adviser would appear to have been present (from either or both of the British Medical Association and BAPIO – the British Association of Physicians of Indian Origin).

At roughly the same time, Lancashire police receive an anonymous allegation of racism directed against myself.

December 2014/early 2015. Mr Peter Read begins to suffer from sepsis and waits several days for emergency surgery, dying on ICU in early 2015.

Early 2015. Two long-standing colleagues resign and UHMBT organises a team of visiting clinical psychologists to visit and counsel the urology department on issues relating to interpersonal relationships and patient care. We all formally commit to respecting both each other and the patients, and to coming together as a team.

Late March 2015. An abusive and witnessed phone call is made to me from a colleague, just days after the psychology review finishes, resulting in my decision to resign with immediate effect unless changes are made. In response, I am immediately moved from the Royal Lancaster Infirmary to Furness General Hospital to separate me from the individual in question.

May 2015. Peter Read's inquest is held. The department is ordered by the coroner to discuss the case in our M&M (Morbidity and Mortality) meeting and produce a report giving the departmental consensus on whether emergency surgery should have been carried out sooner.

June 2015. Two colleagues disobey the coroner and refuse to allow discussion of the case. The ongoing situation and liaison with the coroner's office is then taken over by the Critical Care Division and UHMBT legal office, who instead organise a RCA (root cause analysis) meeting and report. In a direct contradiction of the coroner's orders, all members of the urology department including the head of department are excluded from the meeting.

Autumn 2015. HM coroner rejects the RCA, threatens two Regulation 28s (a notification of risk to the public), but then goes off sick and never comes back to work. The rejected RCA is left on the record and the incident is not revisited for another five years.

In the meantime, I approach the Care Quality Commission (CQC).

October 2015. The CQC approach UHMBT with my concerns about clinical standards. At the end of the same month, without warning, my earnings are cut by around £4000/month.

November 2015. I am appointed, alongside John Dickinson as joint 'interim' clinical lead of the department, standing on a ticket of improved care, respect for both staff and patients and a return to the standards of the department in the late 2000's.

January 2016. A Royal College of Surgeons inspection takes place, which details problems with the department including both clinical standards and interpersonal relationships.

February 2016. Along with Mr Dickinson, I am demoted from the interim joint clinical lead job and Mr B is appointed in my place. I express my extreme concerns to the then-Medical Director that my position will shortly be made untenable.

March 2016. My £4000/month pay cut continues, and an announcement is made in front of my colleagues that, uniquely within the department, my base hospital will be moved from Lancaster to Barrow. This carries the implication that, under NHS rules and unlike everyone else in the department, the work-related travel time and expenses of commuting between Lancaster and Barrow will be removed from my remuneration, I will lose the lease NHS car that I am using, and will additionally have to work an additional 10 hours per week.

May 2016. I am summoned to see the Medical Director and Clinical Director over issues relating to my whistleblowing, where the prospect of disciplinary action is floated. In the end, the written reprimand never materialises.

June 2016. I am informed that the Critical Care Division will not reimburse me for all of the extra sessional pay that has been deducted from my salary. Furthermore, the critical care division threatens to go back through my previous earnings *recouping monies*. It is not clear just how much of my previous earnings might be *recouped* and, after discussions with the BMA, my GP and occupational health, we all agree that I have been placed in a position where I have no choice but to resign as soon as possible. My resignation goes in on the 7th July 2016.

New evidence has emerged that, on that same day, UHMBT begins immediate formal communications with Capsticks Solicitors over my resignation with the aim of heading off any *risks*, despite later claiming to the employment tribunal that my resignation was regretted and not intentional. The emails detailing this are never seen by the employment tribunal.

August 2016. Representations from both Colin Cutting (consultant colleague) and Belinda Pharoah (my ex manager) to UHMBT executives are made on my behalf, requesting a meeting and pointing out that I have no other job to go to and that my last day of work is looming.

September 2016. UHMBT finally agrees to a meeting, several working days after my resignation becomes absolute. At this point, I am unemployed.

At the meeting, it finally becomes clear that there has been a sustained but covert campaign of vilification, directed at me from behind my back and without giving me any chance to respond.

Late 2016. The BMA and Gateley's solicitors formally take on my case for constructive dismissal for whistleblowing. A formal 'subject access request' is made for all communications featuring my name from the accounts of ex-colleagues and managers. UHMBT make counter-allegations to the employment tribunal implying possible fraud by myself, whilst accidentally admitting having illegally deducted a five-figure sum of money from my salary. Proof of the latter is hastily struck out from the employment tribunal record as being *inadmissible evidence*.

UHMBT continue to defend the case.

After about four months out of work, I finally get a job *on the bank* at an hourly rate, working at Noble's Hospital on the Isle of Man, starting just before Christmas.

Early 2017. The first tranche of correspondence from a legal *subject access request* is returned by UHMBT. It has all been rendered unreadable by excessive redaction (censoring).

I have a meeting with Cat Smith, MP, who strongly advises me of my absolute duty to speak of my concerns to the GMC.

I am offered a longer term locum job on the Isle of Man.

Summer 2017. I am formally appointed to a permanent post on the Isle of Man.

A further formal request goes in to Capsticks Solicitors and UHMBT for formal disclosure of all relevant documents prior to the employment tribunal, scheduled for early 2018.

Early 2018. After more requests for full disclosure, a preliminary employment tribunal hearing chaired by Judge Batten, hears evidence that UHMBT have provided all relevant correspondence between myself, ex-colleagues and managers. Judge Batten orders a further search for information and internal documentation relating to the *avoidable death case* (Mr Peter Read).

April 2018. UHMBT via Capsticks solicitors threaten costs of £108,000 if I do not withdraw the employment tribunal case and agree to a COT3 (a form of gag).

The case goes ahead but, on legal advice, I withdraw a good number of pleadings to try and protect myself and the family from costs.

The case attracts the first media attention.

Summer 2018. At the remedies hearing, a settlement is made of £102,500 in my favour, incorporating both £88,000 compensation and outstanding salary from 2015 to 2016 that had still not been paid.

UHMBT announce that they will pursue costs against me.

I begin to have the first thoughts about writing a book.

Late 2018. UHMBT loses its application for costs. Mr Madhra leaves UHMBT by 'mutual agreement'.

The issues are now receiving significant media attention. Mr Peter Read's family get in touch. I am invited down to a whistle-blower evening reception at Westminster and meet with Tim Farron, MP.

Early 2019. *Whistle in the Wind*'s first draft is completed, but no publishers are interested.

May 2019. I am requested to attend Mr Madhra's MPTS/GMC hearing.

July 2019. *Whistle in the Wind* is self-published.

Summer 2019. A joint letter from four local MP's is sent to Matt Hancock, Secretary of State for Health detailing local concerns about the treatment of whistleblowers and governance in UHMBT.

UHMBT's chair resigns shortly after a rather acrimonious public meeting.

Late 2019. Another Trust Governor's meeting is held, being attended by myself, Peter Read's family and Amy Fenton. Niche are formally appointed as a private, NHS funded investigator.

Early 2020. I have my first meeting with Niche.

Spring 2020. COVID-19 strikes. The Isle of Man locks down and I am unable to continue my once fortnightly weekend trips home to the family.

Noble's Hospital shuts to all but emergency care and surgery and staff are redeployed to cope with the local consequences of the pandemic.

Summer 2020. Isle of Man has, for the moment, beaten the virus and I am allowed to go home for a fortnight of compassionate leave.

Autumn 2020. My first MS Teams interview with Niche Consulting is held. New evidence emerges. Niche rejects my concerns about the validity of the emails.

Winter 2020. I am allowed home on a week of compassionate leave. The Isle of Man remains COVID-free, but with very tight border controls. I ask the Medical Protection Society to get involved in my case. Dr Clare Devlin and solicitor Jane Lang are appointed to assist me. The first thoughts of a second book start to crystallise.

Spring 2021. Another outbreak of COVID-19 locks down the Isle of Man again.

Easter 2021. I am allowed home for nine days of compassionate leave. The first draft of *Smoke and Mirrors* is completed.

Late 2021. *Smoke and Mirrors* is published.

GLOSSARY

AfPP	Association for Perioperative Practice.
APPG	All-Party Parliamentary Groups
BAME	Black, Asian Minority Ethnic
BAPIO	British Association of Physicians of Indian Origin
BMA	British Medical Association
COT3	Legally Binding Agreement to settle actual or potential claims in an employment tribunal
CQC	Care Quality Commission
CT scan	Computerised Tomographic Scan
GMC	General Medical Council
ICU	Intensive Care Unit
M&M	Morbidity and Mortality
MPS	Medical Protection Society
MPTS	Medical Practitioners Tribunal Service
NDA	Non Disclosure Agreement
NHS	National Health Service
PALS	Patient Advice and Liaison Service
PIDA	Public Interest Disclosure Act
Protect	Whistleblowing Charity (formerly Public Concern at Work)
RCA	Root Cause Analysis
RTX	Unique UHMBT Patient identity hospital number
SRA	Solicitors Regulatory Authority
TTO	To take out
UHMBT/MBHT	University Hospitals of Morecambe Bay Trust

Printed in Great Britain
by Amazon